This report contains the collective views of an international group of experts and does not necessarily represent the decisions or the stated policy of the United Nations Environment Programme, the International Labour Organisation, or the World Health Organization

Environmental Health Criteria 94

PERMETHRIN

Published under the joint sponsorship of
the United Nations Environment Programme,
the International Labour Organisation,
and the World Health Organization

World Health Organization
Geneva, 1990

The **International Programme on Chemical Safety (IPCS)** is a joint venture of the United Nations Environment Programme, the International Labour Organisation, and the World Health Organization. The main objective of the IPCS is to carry out and disseminate evaluations of the effects of chemicals on human health and the quality of the environment. Supporting activities include the development of epidemiological, experimental laboratory, and risk-assessment methods that could produce internationally comparable results, and the development of manpower in the field of toxicology. Other activities carried out by the IPCS include the development of know-how for coping with chemical accidents, coordination of laboratory testing and epidemiological studies, and promotion of research on the mechanisms of the biological action of chemicals.

WHO Library Cataloguing in Publication Data

Permethrin.

(Environmental health criteria ; 94)

1. Pyrethrins. I. Series

ISBN 92 4 154294 2 (NLM Classification: WA 240)
ISSN 0250-863X

The designations employed and the presentation of the material in this publication do not imply the expression of any opinion whatsoever on the part of the Secretariat of the World Health Organization concerning the legal status of any country, territory, city, or area or of its authorities, or concerning the delimitation of its frontiers or boundaries.

The mention of specific companies or of certain manufacturers' products does not imply that they are endorsed or recommended by the World Health Organization in preference to others of a similar nature that are not mentioned. Errors and omissions excepted, the names of proprietary products are distinguished by initial capital letters.

Printed in Finland
DHSS — Vammala — 5000

CONTENTS

ENVIRONMENTAL HEALTH CRITERIA FOR PERMETHRIN

INTRODUCTION 11

1. SUMMARY, EVALUATION, CONCLUSIONS, AND RECOMMENDATION 13

1.1 Summary and evaluation 13
1.1.1 Identity, physical and chemical properties, analytical methods 13
1.1.2 Production and use 13
1.1.3 Human exposure 13
1.1.4 Environmental fate 14
1.1.5 Kinetics and metabolism 14
1.1.6 Effects on organisms in the environment 14
1.1.7 Effects on experimental animals and *in vitro* test systems 15
1.1.8 Effects on human beings 16
1.2 Conclusions 17
1.2.1 General population 17
1.2.2 Occupational exposure 17
1.2.3 Environment 17
1.3 Recommendations 17

2. IDENTITY, PHYSICAL AND CHEMICAL PROPERTIES, ANALYTICAL METHODS 18

2.1 Chemical identity 18
2.2 Physical and chemical properties 21
2.3 Analytical methods 21

3. SOURCES OF HUMAN AND ENVIRONMENTAL EXPOSURE; ENVIRONMENTAL LEVELS 25

3.1 Industrial production 25
3.2 Use pattern 25
3.3 Residues in food and other products 26
3.4 Residues in the environment 28

4. ENVIRONMENTAL TRANSPORT, DISTRIBUTION, AND TRANSFORMATION 29

4.1 Transport and distribution between media 29
4.2 Photodecomposition 32
4.3 Degradation in plants 33
4.4 Degradation in soils 34

5. KINETICS AND METABOLISM 38

5.1 Metabolism in mammals 38
5.1.1 Mouse 38
5.1.2 Rat 38
5.1.3 Goat 41
5.1.4 Cow 41
5.1.5 Man 42
5.2 Metabolism in hens 42
5.3 Enzymatic systems for biotransformation 44

6. EFFECTS ON THE ENVIRONMENT 46

6.1 Toxicity to aquatic organisms 46
6.1.1 Aquatic microorganisms 46
6.1.2 Aquatic invertebrates 46
6.1.3 Fish 47
6.1.4 Field studies and community effects 48
6.2 Toxicity to terrestrial organisms 55
6.2.1 Soil microorganisms 55
6.2.2 Terrestrial invertebrates 55
6.2.3 Birds 59
6.2.4 Mammals 59
6.3 Uptake, loss, bioaccumulation, and biomagnification 60

7. EFFECTS ON EXPERIMENTAL ANIMALS AND *IN VITRO* TEST SYSTEMS 63

7.1 Acute toxicity 63
7.2 Subacute and subchronic toxicity 67
7.2.1 Oral exposure 67
7.2.1.1 Mouse 67
7.2.1.2 Rat 68
7.2.1.3 Dog 70
7.2.1.4 Rabbit 71
7.2.1.5 Cow 71
7.2.2 Dermal exposure 71
7.2.3 Inhalation exposure 72
7.3 Primary irritation 73
7.3.1 Skin irritation 73
7.3.2 Eye irritation 73
7.4 Sensitization 73
7.5 Long-term toxicity 74
7.5.1 Mouse 74
7.5.2 Rat 75
7.6 Carcinogenesis 76
7.6.1 Mouse 76
7.6.1.1 ICI study 76
7.6.1.2 FMC II study 77

7.6.1.3 BW study 77
7.6.1.4 Appraisal of mouse studies on carcinogenicity 77
7.6.2 Rat 79
7.6.2.1 ICI study 79
7.6.2.2 BW study 79
7.6.2.3 Appraisal of rat studies on carcinogenicity 79
7.7 Mutagenicity 80
7.7.1 Microorganism and insects 80
7.7.2 Mammals 80
7.8 Teratogenicity and reproduction studies 81
7.8.1 Teratogenicity studies 81
7.8.1.1 Mouse 81
7.8.1.2 Rat 81
7.8.1.3 Rabbit 83
7.8.2 Reproduction studies 83
7.8.2.1 Rat 83
7.9 Neurotoxicity 84
7.9.1 Rat 84
7.9.2 Hen 85
7.10 Behavioural effects 86
7.11 Miscellaneous studies 86
7.12 Mechanism of toxicity (mode of action) 87

8. EFFECTS ON HUMANS 89

8.1 Occupational exposure 89
8.2 Clinical studies 90

9. PREVIOUS EVALUATIONS BY INTERNATIONAL BODIES 92

REFERENCES 93

APPENDIX I 115

FRENCH TRANSLATION OF SUMMARY, EVALUATION, CONCLUSIONS, AND RECOMMENDATIONS 120

WHO TASK GROUP ON ENVIRONMENTAL HEALTH CRITERIA FOR PERMETHRIN

Members

Dr V. Benes, Department of Toxicology and Reference Laboratory, Institute of Hygiene and Epidemiology, Prague, Czechoslovakia

Dr S. Dobson, Institute of Terrestrial Ecology, Monks Wood Experimental Station, Huntingdon, United Kingdom

Dr Y. Hayashi, Division of Pathology, National Institute of Hygienic Sciences, Tokyo, Japan

Dr S. Johnson, Hazard Evaluation Division, Office of Pesticide Programme, US Environmental Protection Agency, Washington DC, USA (*Chairman*)

Dr S.K. Kashyap, National Institute of Occupational Health (ICMR) Ahmedabad, India (*Vice-Chairman*)

Dr Yu. I. Kundiev, Research Institute of Labour, Hygiene, and Occupational Diseases, Kiev, USSR

Dr J.P. Leahey, ICI Agrochemicals, Jealotts Hill Research Station, Bracknell, United Kingdom (*Rapporteur*)

Dr J. Miyamoto, Takarazuka Research Centre, Sumitomo Chemical Company, Takarazuka, Hyogo, Japan

Dr Y. Takenaka, Division of Information on Chemical Safety, National Institute of Hygienic Sciences, Tokyo, Japan

Representatives of Other Organizations

Dr M. Ikeda, International Commission on Occupational Health. Department of Environmental Health, Tohoku University, School of Medicine, Sendai, Japan

Dr H. Naito, World Federation of Poison Control Centres and Clinical Toxicology. Institute of Clinical Medicine, University of Tsukuba, Tsukuba-Shi, Ibaraki, Japan

Observers

Dr M. Matsuo, Sumitomo Chemical Company, Biochemistry & Toxicology Laboratory, Osaka, Japan

Dr Y. Okuno, Sumitomo Chemical Company, Biochemistry & Toxicology Laboratory, Osaka, Japan

Dr N. Punja, International Group of National Association of Manufacturers of Agrochemical Products (GIFAP), ICI Plant Protection Division, Fenhurst, Haslemere, United Kingdom

Secretariat

Dr K.W. Jager, International Programme on Chemical Safety, World Health Organization, Geneva, Switzerland (*Secretary*)

Dr R. Plestina, Division of Vector Control, Delivery and Management of Vector Control, World Health Organization, Geneva, Switzerland

Dr J. Sekizawa, Section of Information and Investigation, Division of Information on Chemical Safety, National Institute of Hygienic Sciences, Tokyo, Japan (*Rapporteur*)

NOTE TO READERS OF THE CRITERIA DOCUMENTS

Every effort has been made to present information in the criteria documents as accurately as possible without unduly delaying their publication. In the interest of all users of the environmental health criteria documents, readers are kindly requested to communicate any errors that may have occurred to the Manager of the International Programme on Chemical Safety, World Health Organization, Geneva, Switzerland, in order that they may be included in corrigenda, which will appear in subsequent volumes.

* * *

A detailed data profile and a legal file can be obtained from the International Register of Potentially Toxic Chemicals, Palais des Nations, 1211 Geneva 10, Switzerland (Telephone No. 7988400 or 7985850).

* * *

The proprietary information contained in this document cannot replace documentation for registration purposes, because the latter has to be closely linked to the source, the manufacturing route and the purity/impurities of the substance to be registered. The data should be used in accordance with paragraphs 82-84 and recommendations paragraph 90 of the Second FAO Government Consultation (FAO, 1982).

ENVIRONMENTAL HEALTH CRITERIA FOR PERMETHRIN

A WHO Task Group on Environmental Health Criteria for Fenvalerate, Permethrin, and d-Phenothrin met in Tokyo from 4 to 8 July 1988. This meeting was convened with the financial assistance of the Ministry of Health and Welfare, Tokyo, Japan, and was hosted by the National Institute of Hygienic Sciences (NIHS) in Tokyo.

Dr T. Furukawa and Dr K. Shirota opened the meeting on behalf of the Ministry of Health and Welfare, and Dr A. Tanimura, Director-General of the NIHS welcomed the participants to the Institute. Dr M. Mercier, Manager of the International Programme on Chemical Safety, welcomed the participants on behalf of the three IPCS cooperating organizations (UNEP/ILO/WHO). The group reviewed and revised the draft monograph and made an evaluation of the risks for human health and the environment from exposure to permethrin.

The first draft of this document was prepared by DR J. MIYAMOTO and DR M. MATSUO of Sumitomo Chemical Company with the assistance of the staff of the National Institute of Hygienic Sciences, Tokyo, Japan. Dr I. Yamamoto of the Tokyo University of Agriculture and Dr M. Eto of Kyushu University, Japan, assisted with the finalization of the draft. The second draft was prepared by DR J. SEKIZAWA, NIHS, Tokyo, incorporating comments received following circulation of the first draft to the IPCS contact points for Environmental Health Criteria documents. Dr K.W. Jager and Dr P.G. Jenkins, both members of the IPCS Central Unit, were responsible for the technical development and editing, respectively, of this monograph.

The assistance of the Sumitomo Chemical Company, Japan, and ICI Agrochemicals, United Kingdom, in making available to the IPCS and the Task Group their toxicological proprietary information on permethrin is gratefully acknowledged. This allowed the Task Group to make its evaluation on the basis of more complete data.

* * *

The United Kingdom Department of Health and Social Security generously supported the cost of printing.

ABBREVIATIONS

ai	active ingredient
Cl_2CA	3-(2,2-dichlorovinyl)-2,2-dimethylcyclopropanecarboxyclic acid
ECG	electrocardiogram
EEG	electroencephalogram
FID	flame ionization detector
GC	gas chromatography
GC-ECD	gas chromatography with electron capture detector
GC-SIM	gas chromatography with selected ion monitoring
GLC	gas-liquid chromatography
HPLC	high-performance liquid chromatography
JMPR	Joint FAO/WHO Meeting on Pesticide Residues
NOEL	no-observed-effect level
PBacid	3-phenoxybenzoic acid
PBalc	3-phenoxybenzyl alcohol
PBald	3-phenoxybenzaldehyde
TLC	thin-layer chromatography

INTRODUCTION

SYNTHETIC PYRETHROIDS - A PROFILE

1. During investigations to modify the chemical structures of natural pyrethrins, a certain number of synthetic pyrethroids were produced with improved physical and chemical properties and greater biological activity. Several of the earlier synthetic pyrethroids were successfully commercialized, mainly for the control of household insects. Other more recent pyrethroids have been introduced as agricultural insecticides because of their excellent activity against a wide range of insect pests and their non-persistence in the environment.

2. The pyrethroids constitute another group of insecticides in addition to organochlorine, organophosphorus, carbamate, and other compounds. Pyrethroids commercially available to date include allethrin, resmethrin, d-phenothrin, and tetramethrin (for insects of public health importance), and cypermethrin, deltamethrin, fenvalerate, and permethrin (mainly for agricultural insects). Other pyrethroids are also available including furamethrin, kadethrin, and tellallethrin (usually for household insects), fenpropathrin, tralomethrin, cyhalothrin, lambda-cyhalothrin, tefluthrin, cyfluthrin, flucythrinate, fluvalinate, and biphenate (for agricultural insects).

3. Toxicological evaluations of several synthetic pyrethroids have been performed by the FAO/WHO Joint Meeting on Pesticide Residues (JMPR). The acceptable daily intake (ADI) has been estimated by the JMPR for cypermethrin, deltamethrin, fenvalerate, permethrin, d-phenothrin, cyfluthrin, cyhalothrin, and flucythrinate.

4. Chemically, synthetic pyrethroids are esters of specific acids (e.g., chrysanthemic acid, halo-substituted chrysanthemic acid, 2-(4-chlorophenyl)-3-methylbutyric acid) and alcohols (e.g., allethrolone, 3-phenoxybenzyl alcohol). For certain pyrethroids, asymmetric centre(s) exist in the acid and/or alcohol moiety, and the commercial products sometimes consist of a mixture of both optical (1R/1S or d/l) and geometric (cis/trans) isomers. However, most of the insecticidal activity of such products may reside in only one or two isomers. Some of the products (e.g., d-phenothrin, deltamethrin) consist only of such active isomer(s).

5. Synthetic pyrethroids are neuropoisons acting on the axons in the peripheral and central nervous systems by interacting with sodium channels in mammals and/or insects. A single dose produces toxic signs in mammals, such as tremors, hyperexcitability, salivation, choreoathetosis, and paralysis. The signs disappear fairly rapidly, and the animals recover, generally within a week. At near-

lethal dose levels, synthetic pyrethroids cause transient changes in the nervous system, such as axonal swelling and/or breaks and myelin degeneration in sciatic nerves. They are not considered to cause delayed neurotoxicity of the kind induced by some organophosphorus compounds. The mechanism of toxicity of synthetic pyrethroids and their classification into two types are discussed in the Appendix.

6. Some pyrethroids (e.g., deltamethrin, fenvalerate, cyhalothrin, lambda-cyhalothrin, flucythrinate, and cypermethrin) may cause a transient itching and/or burning sensation in exposed human skin.

7. Synthetic pyrethroids are generally metabolized in mammals through ester hydrolysis, oxidation, and conjugation, and there is no tendency to accumulate in tissues. In the environment, synthetic pyrethroids are fairly rapidly degraded in soil and in plants. Ester hydrolysis and oxidation at various sites on the molecule are the major degradation processes. The pyrethroids are strongly adsorbed on soil and sediments, and hardly eluted with water. There is little tendency for bioaccumulation in organisms.

8. Because of low application rates and rapid degradation in the environment, residues in food are generally low.

9. Synthetic pyrethroids have been shown to be toxic for fish, aquatic arthropods, and honey bees in laboratory tests. But, in practical usage, no serious adverse effects have been noticed because of the low rates of application and lack of persistence in the environment. The toxicity of synthetic pyrethroids in birds and domestic animals is low.

10. In addition to the evaluation documents of FAO/WHO, there are several good reviews and books on the chemistry, metabolism, mammalian toxicity, environmental effects, etc. of synthetic pyrethroids, including those by Elliott (1977), Miyamoto (1981), Miyamoto & Kearney (1983), and Leahey (1985).

1. SUMMARY AND EVALUATION, CONCLUSIONS, RECOMMENDATION

1.1 Summary and Evaluation

1.1.1 Identity, physical and chemical properties, analytical methods

Permethrin was first synthesized in 1973 and marketed in 1977 as a photostable pyrethroid. It is an ester of the dichloro analogue of chrysanthemic acid, 3-(2,2-dichlorovinyl)-2,2-dimethylcyclopropane-carboxylic acid (Cl_2CA), and 3-phenoxybenzyl alcohol. Technical products are a mixture of four stereoisomers with the configurations [1R,trans], [1R,cis], [1S,trans], and [1S,cis] in the approximate ratio of 3:2:3:2. The ratio of cis:trans is around 2:3 and 1R:1S is 1:1 (racemic). The [1R,cis] isomer is the most insecticidally active of the isomers, followed by the [1R,trans] isomer.

Technical grade permethrin is a brown or yellowish brown liquid which may crystallize partly at room temperature. The melting point is approximately 35°C and the boiling point is 220°C at 0.05 mmHg. The specific gravity is 1.214 at 25°C and the vapour pressure is 1.3 μPa at 20°C. Permethrin is almost insoluble in water (0.2 mg/litre at 30°C), but is soluble in organic solvents such as acetone, hexane, and xylene. It is stable to light and heat, but unstable in alkaline media.

Residue and environmental analyses are performed using a gas chromatograph equipped with an electron capture detector (minimum detectable concentration of 0.005 mg/kg). Technical products are analysed using a gas chromatograph with a flame ionization detector.

1.1.2 Production and use

Approximately 600 tonnes per year of permethrin is at present used world-wide, mostly for agricultural purposes. It has a potential application in the protection of stored grain and it has been used in aerial application for forest protection and vector control, for the control of noxious insects in the household and on cattle, for the control of body lice, and in mosquito nets.

Permethrin is formulated as emulsifiable concentrate, ultra-low-volume concentrate, wettable powder, and dustable powder.

1.1.3 Human exposure

The rate of decline of residue levels in various crops is fairly slow, half-lives ranging from about 1 to 3 weeks depending on the crop. However, when permethrin is used as recommended, there is no significant increase in residues following repeated application.

Exposure of the general population to permethrin is mainly via dietary residues. Residue levels in crops grown according to good agricultural practice are generally low. The resulting exposure of the general population is expected to be low, but precise data in the form of total-diet studies is lacking.

Information on occupational exposure to permethrin is very limited.

1.1.4 Environmental fate

In laboratory studies, permethrin has been shown to degrade in soil with a half-life of 28 days or less. The trans isomer degraded more rapidly than the cis isomer, ester cleavage being the major initial degradative reaction. The compounds generated by ester cleavage were then further oxidised, eventually yielding carbon dioxide as the major terminal product. Studies to investigate the leaching potential of permethrin and its degradates showed that very little downward movement occurs in soil.

Permethrin deposited on plants degrades with a half-life of approximately 10 days. Ester cleavage and conjugation of the acid and alcohol released is the major degradation pathway. Hydroxylation at various positions of the molecule and photo-induced cis-trans interconversion also occur.

In water and on soil surfaces permethrin is photodegraded by sunlight. Ester cleavage and cis-trans interconversion are, as with plants, the major reactions.

In general, the degradative processes which occur in the environment lead to less toxic products.

Permethrin disappears rapidly from the environment, in 6-24 h from ponds and streams, 7 days from pond sediment, and 58 days from foliage and soil in a forest. From cotton leaves in a field, 30% of the compound was lost within 1 week.

Under aerobic conditions in soil, permethrin degrades with a half-life of 28 days.

There is very little movement of permethrin in the environment, and it is unlikely that it will attain significant levels in the environment.

1.1.5 Kinetics and metabolism

Permethrin administered to mammals was rapidly metabolized and almost completely excreted in urine and faeces within 12 days. The trans isomer, being much more susceptible to esterase attack than the cis isomer, was eliminated faster than the cis isomer. The major metabolic reactions were ester cleavage and oxidation, particularly at the terminal aromatic ring of the phenoxybenzyl moiety and the geminal dimethyl group of the cyclopropane ring, followed by conjugation. Less than 0.7% of the dose was detected in the milk of goats or cows administered permethrin orally.

1.1.6 Effects on organisms in the environment

In laboratory tests, permethrin has been shown to be highly toxic for aquatic arthropods, LC_{50} values ranging from 0.018 μg/litre for larval stone crabs to 1.26 μg/litre for a cladoceran. It is also highly toxic for fish, with 96-h LC_{50} values ranging from 0.62 μg/litre for larval rainbow trout to 314 μg/litre for adult rainbow trout. The no-observed-effect level for early life stages of the sheepshead minnow over 28 days is 10 μg/litre and the chronic no-effect level for fathead minnow is 0.66-1.4 μg/litre. Permethrin is less toxic to aquatic molluscs and amphibia, 96-h LC_{50} values being >1000 μg/litre and 7000 μg/litre, respectively.

In field tests and in the use of the compound under practical conditions, this high potential toxicity is not manifested. An extensive literature exists on the effects of using permethrin in agriculture, forestry, and in vector control in many parts of the world. Some aquatic arthropods are killed, particularly when water is over-sprayed but the effects on populations of organisms is temporary. There have been no reports of fish killed in the field. This reduced toxicity in the field is related to the strong adsorption of the compound to sediments and its rapid degradation. Sediment-bound permethrin is toxic to burrowing organisms but this effect also is temporary.

Permethrin is highly toxic for honey bees. The topical LD_{50} is 0.11 μg/bee, but there is a strong repellent effect of permethrin to bees which reduced the toxic effect in practice. There is no evidence for significant kills of honey bees under normal use. Permethrin is more toxic to predator mites than to the target pest species.

Permethrin has very low toxicity to birds when given orally or fed in the diet. The LD_{50} is >3000 mg/kg body weight for acute single oral dosage and for dietary exposure it is >5000 mg/kg diet. It has no effect on reproduction in the hen at a dose of 40 mg/kg diet.

Permethrin is readily taken up by aquatic organisms, bioconcentration factors ranging from 43 to 750 for various organisms. In all the aquatic organisms studied, absorbed permethrin is rapidly lost on transfer to clean water. There is no bioaccumulation in birds. The compound can, therefore, be regarded as having no tendency to bioaccumulate in practice.

1.1.7 Effects on experimental animals and in vitro test systems

Permethrin has a low acute toxicity to rats, mice, rabbits, and guinea-pigs, though the LD_{50} value varies considerably according to the vehicle used and the cis:trans isomeric ratio. Signs of acute poisoning become apparent within 2 h of dosing and persist for up to 3 days. [1R,*cis*]- and [1R,*trans*]-permethrin belong to the type I group of pyrethroids, which typically cause tremor (T-syndrome), incoordination, hyperactivity, prostration, and paralysis. Core temperature is markedly increased during poisoning.

None of the metabolites of permethrin shows a higher acute (oral or intraperitoneal) toxicity than permethrin itself.

Permethrin caused a mild primary irritation of the intact and abraded skin of rabbits but did not cause a photochemical irritation reaction after exposure of treated areas of rabbit skin to ultra-violet light. Permethrin did not cause a sensitization reaction in guinea-pigs.

Oral subacute and subchronic toxicity studies of permethrin have been performed in rats and mice at dose levels up to 10 000 mg/kg diet and for 14 days to 26 weeks in duration. Changes detected at the higher level were an increase in liver/body weight ratio, hypertrophy in the liver, and clinical signs of poisoning such as tremor. The no-observed-effects levels (NOEL) in rats ranged from 20 mg/kg diet (in studies lasting 90 days or 6 months) to 1500 mg/kg diet (in a 6-month study).

NOEL values in dogs ranged from 5 mg/kg body weight in 3-month studies to 250 mg/kg body weight in 6-month studies.

In long-term studies in mice and rats, an increase in liver weight was found which was considered to be associated with an induction of the liver microsomal enzyme system.

The NOEL in a 2-year rat study was 100 mg/kg diet, corresponding to 5.0 mg/kg body weight.

There were indications, from three long-term mouse studies, of oncogenicity in the lungs of one strain of mouse (females only) at the highest dose level (5 g/kg diet). Studies in rats revealed no oncogenic potential in either sex.

Permethrin was not mutagenic in *in vivo* or *in vitro* studies.

Toxicological evidence from mutagenicity studies and from long-term mouse and rat studies suggests that permethrin's oncogenic potential is very low, is limited to female mice, and is probably epigenetic.

Permethrin is not teratogenic to rats, mice, or rabbits at dose levels up to 225, 150, and 1800 mg/kg body weight, respectively.

In a 3-generation reproduction study, permethrin did not induce adverse effects at levels up to 2500 mg/kg diet.

Permethrin fed to rats at high dose levels (6600-7000 mg/kg diet) for 14 days induced sciatic nerve damage in one study but did not produce any ultrastructural changes in the sciatic nerve in another study. Permethrin did not cause delayed neurotoxicity in hens.

1.1.8 Effects on human beings

Permethrin can induce skin sensations and paraesthesia in exposed workers, which develop after a latent period of approximately 30 min, peak by 8 h and disappear within 24 h. Numbness, itching, tingling, and burning are symptoms frequently reported.

No poisoning cases have been reported.

The likelihood of oncogenic effects in human beings is extremely low or non-existent.

There are no indications that permethrin has an adverse effect on human beings when used as recommended.

1.2 Conclusions

1.2.1 General population

The exposure of the general population to permethrin is expected to be low. It is not likely to present a hazard provided it is used as recommended.

1.2.2 Occupational exposure

With reasonable work practices, hygiene measures, and safety precautions, permethrin is unlikely to present a hazard to those exposed occupationally.

1.2.3 Environment

It is unlikely that permethrin or its degradation products will attain levels of environmental significance provided that recommended application rates are used. Under laboratory conditions permethrin is highly toxic to fish, aquatic anthropods, and honey bees. However, lasting adverse effects are not likely to occur under field conditions provided it is used as recommended.

1.3 Recommendations

Although dietary levels arising from recommended usage are considered to be low, confirmation of this through inclusion of permethrin in monitoring studies should be considered.

No adverse effects have been reported following human exposure to permethrin during the many years of its use. Nevertheless, it would be wise to maintain observations of human exposure.

2. IDENTITY, PHYSICAL AND CHEMICAL PROPERTIES, ANALYTICAL METHODS

2.1 Chemical Identity

Permethrin was synthesized as one of the new photostable pyrethroids by Elliott et al. (1973). It is prepared by the esterification of the dichloro analogue of chrysanthemic acid, i.e. (1R,*cis*; 1R,*trans*; 1S,*cis*; 1S,*trans*)-3-(2,2-dichlorovinyl)-2,2-dimethyl-cyclopropanecarboxyclic acid (Cl_2CA), with 3-phenoxybenzyl alcohol (PBalc). It contains four stereoisomers due to the chirality of the cyclopropane ring (Fig.1). The cis:trans isomer ratio is reported to be 2:3 and the optical ratio of 1R:1S is 1:1 (racemic) (FAO/WHO, 1980b). Thus, permethrin contains the [1R,trans], [1R,cis], [1S,trans], and [1S,cis] isomers in the approximate ratio of 3:2:3:2. Table 1 gives further details of the chemical identity of permethrin.

The [1R,cis] isomer is the most insecticidally active among the isomers, followed by the [1R,trans] isomer.

Molecular formula: $C_{21}H_{20}Cl_2O_3$

Chemical formula:

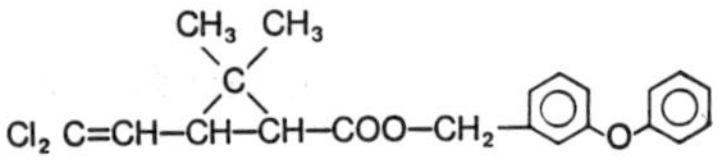

Chemical structures of 4 stereoisomers:

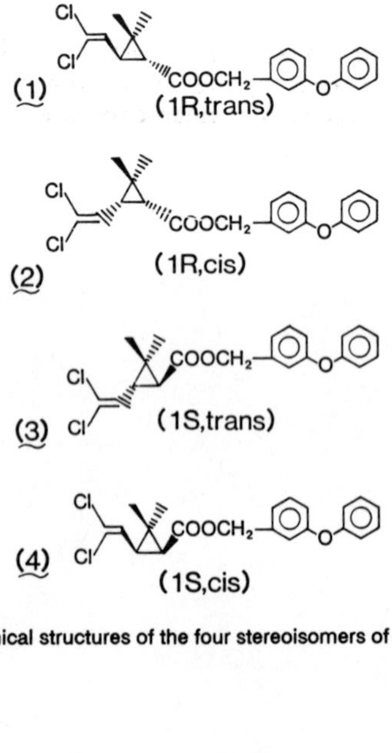

Fig. 1. Chemical structures of the four stereoisomers of permethrin

Table 1. Chemical identity of permethrin and its various stereoisomeric compositions

Common name/ CAS Registry No./ NIOSH Accession No.[a]	CAS Index name (9CI) Stereospecific name[b]	Stereoisomeric composition[c]	Synonyms and trade names
Permethrin 52645-53-1 GZ1255000	Cyclopropanecarboxylic acid, 3-(2,2-dichloroethenyl)-2,2-dimethyl-, (3-phenoxyphenyl)methyl ester 3-Phenoxybenzyl (1RS,*cis*,*trans*)-3-(2,2-dichlorovinyl)-2,2-dimethyl-cyclopropanecarboxylate	(1):(2):(3):(4) =3:2:3:2	Permethrina, Ambush, Pounce, Outflank, Extin, Ectiban, Stockade, NRDC143, FMC33297, S-3151, SBP-1513, PP557, A13-29158, BW-21-Z
(+)-*cis*-Permethrin 54774-45-7 GZ1257000	same as permethrin 3-Phenoxybenzyl (1R,*cis*)-3-(2,2-dichlorovinyl)-2,2-dimethyl-cyclopropanecarboxylate	-	-
Permethrin (racemic mixture) - GZ1261000	same as permethrin 3-Phenoxybenzyl (1R,*cis*,*trans*)-3-(2,2-dichlorovinyl)-2,2-dimethyl-cyclopropanecarboxylate	*cis*:*trans* = 2:3	-
(+)-*trans*-Permethrin 51877-74-8 GZ1260000	same as permethrin 3-Phenoxybenzyl (1R,*trans*)-3-(2,2-dichlorovinyl)-2,2-dimethyl-cyclopropanecarboxylate	-	-

Table 1 (contd).

Common name/ CAS Registry No./ NIOSH Accession No.[a]	CAS Index name (9CI) Stereospecific name[b]	Stereoisomeric composition[c]	Synonyms and trade names
cis-Permethrin 61949-76-6 GZ1251540	same as permethrin 3-Phenoxybenzyl (1RS,*cis*)-3-(2,2-dichlorovinyl)-2,2-dimethyl-cyclopropanecarboxylate	-	-

a Registry of Toxic Effects of Chemical Substances (RTECS) (1981-1982 edition).
b (1R), (+) or (1S), (-) in the acid part of permethrin signifies the same stereospecific conformation, respectively.
c Numbers in parentheses identify the structures shown in Fig. 1.

2.2 Physical and Chemical Properties

The physical and chemical properties of technical permethrin (cis/trans isomeric ratio = 40:60, purity not less than 89%) are summarized in Table 2. Permethrin is stable to heat and light. It is more resistant in acidic media than alkaline, with an optimum stability at pH 4.

Table 2. Physicochemical properties of technical permethrin[a]

Physical state	crystal or viscous liquid
Colour	yellow brown to brown
Relative molecular mass	391.31
Melting point	34 - 39 °C 63 - 65 °C (cis); 44 - 47 °C (trans)
Boiling point	220 °C (6.67 Pa), 200 °C (1.33 Pa)
Water solubility (30 °C)	0.2 mg/litre
Solubility in organic solvents (25 °C)	soluble or miscible with most organic solvents: acetone (450 g/litre), hexane (> 1 kg/kg), methanol (258 g/kg), xylene ($\geq$ 1 kg/kg)
Density (25 °C)	1.214
Vapor pressure (20 °C)	Technical grade : 1.3 μPa Pure : 2.5 μPa (cis), 1.5 μPa (trans)
Octanol-water partition coefficient (log P_{ow})	6.5[b]

[a] From: Meister et al. (1983); Worthing & Walker (1987); FAO/WHO (1980b); Wells et al. (1986)
[b] From: Schimmel et al. (1983)

2.3 Analytical Methods

Methods for the analysis of permethrin are summarized in Table 3. The common procedure of residue and environmental analysis consists of (a) extraction, (b) partition, (c) chromatographic separation (clean up), and (d) quantitative and qualitative analysis of the insecticide by analytical instruments. Table 3 also indicates minimum detectable concentration (MDC) and percentage recovery.

To analyse technical grade permethrin, the product is dissolved in chloroform, together with dioctyl phthalate (as an internal standard), and the solution is injected into a GLC system equipped with flame ionization detector (FID) (Horiba et al., 1977).

The Joint FAO/WHO Codex Alimentarius Committee has published recommendations for methods of analysis of permethrin residues (FAO/WHO, 1985c).

In the internationally accepted CIPAC (Collaborative International Pesticide Analytical Council) method for permethrin analysis, the product is dissolved in 4-methylpentan-2-one containing *n*-octacosane as internal standard. Separation is carried out by GLC on a column of chromosorb W-HP coated with silicone OV 210 (Henriet et al., 1985).

A gas chromatographic method for determining permethrin in technical and formulated products has been developed and subjected to a collaborative study involving 19 laboratories (Tyler, 1987). The column used was a 1.0 m x 4 mm glass column packed with 3% OV-210 on chromosorb W-HP. When five samples of technical material (90-95%), eight of emulsifiable concentrates (10-50%), two of wettable powders (20-30%), one of dustable powder (1-2%), and one of water-dispersible granules (1-2%) were analysed, the coefficient of variation of the results obtained ranged from 0.79 to 4.24%. The method was adopted as an official first-action method by the Association of Official Analytical Chemists.

Table 3. Analytical methods for permethrin

Sample	Sample preparation				Determination GLC or HPLC; detector,[b] carrier, flow, column, temperature, retention time	MDC[c]	% Recovery (fortification level) (mg/litre)[d]	Reference
	Extraction solvent	Partition	Clean up Column	Elution				
Residue analysis								
apple	*n*-hexane/ acetone : (1/1)	ext.sol.[a] /H_2O	Silica gel	CH_2Cl_2	ECD-GC,N_2, 50 ml/min, 1 m, 3% OV-7, 235 °C	0.01	91 - 106 (0.1 - 1.0)	Baker & Bottomley (1982)
pear	*n*-hexane/ acetone : (1/1)	ext.sol.[a] /H_2O	Silica gel	CH_2Cl_2	HPLC UV-206 nm, 25 cm ODS, propan-2-o1, 1 ml/min	0.05	81 - 95 (0.1 - 1.0)	Baker & Bottomley (1982)
blueberry	acetone	*n*-hexane/ sat.NaCl	Florisil	benzene/ *n*-hexane (4/1)	ECD-GC, N_2, 60 ml/min, 0.9 m, 3% OV-210, 200 °C, 7.0(cis), 8.3 (trans) min	0.01	cis:79.6 - 87.1 (0.05 - 0.25) trans:73.3 - 84.2 (0.05 - 0.25)	MacPhee et al. (1982)
celery	CH_3CN	*n*-hexane/ 2% NaCl	Florisil	CH_3CN/ CH_2Cl_2/ *n*-hexane (0.35/50/50)	ECD-GC, N_2, 100 ml/min 1.8 m, Ultra-Bond 20M, 220 °C, 3.5, 4.1 min	0.005	94.2 - 97.0 (0.01 - 1.0)	Braun & Stanek (1982)
corn	pentane	CH_3CN/ pentane	Alumina	pentane/ ethyl acetate (97/3)	FID-GC, N_2, 28 ml/min 1.22 m, 5% OV-225, 250 °C, 9.5(cis), 10.0 (trans) min	0.2	87.5 - 105 (0.2 - 22)	Simonaitis & Cail (1977)

Table 3 (contd).

Sample	Extraction solvent	Sample preparation: Partition	Clean up: Column	Clean up: Elution	Determination GLC or HPLC; detector,[b] carrier, flow, column, temperature, retention time	MDC[c]	% Recovery (fortification level) (mg/litre)[d]	Reference
Residue analysis (contd).								
beef muscle	CH_3CN/ H_2O (85/15)	*n*-hexane 2% NaCl	Florisil	CH_3CN/ CH_2Cl_2/ *n*-hexane (0.35/50/50)	ECD-GC, N_2, 100 ml/min 1.8 m, Ultra-Bond 20M, 220 °C, 3.5(cis), 4.1 (trans) min	0.005	82.9 - 89.9 (0.01 - 1.0)	Braun & Stanek (1982)
Environmental analysis								
waste water	XAD-2 resin, ether		Florisil	*n*-hexane /ether (9/1)	GC-SIM/MS, He, 25 ml/min, 1.8 m, SP-2250, 230 °C, 3.5(cis), 3.7 (trans) min	50 ng/litre	95 (0.11) 95 (0.26)	Siegel et al. (1980)
runoff (sediment +water)	*n*-hexane				ECD-GC, N_2, 150 ml/min, 0.91 m, 5% SP-2330, 215 °C, 3(cis), 4 (trans) min	100 ng/litre	97	Carroll et al. (1981)
Product analysis								
technical grade	$CHCl_3$				FID-GC, N_2, 40 ml/min, 2% LAC-2R-446, 200 °C			Horiba et al. (1977)

a ext. sol = extraction solvent.
b detector (ECD-GC = Coulson electrolytic conductivity detector-GC; GC-SIM/MS = GC-selected ion monitoring with mass spectroscopy).
c MDC = minimum detectable concentration (mg/kg, unless stated otherwise).
d fortification level indicates the concentration of permethrin added to control samples for the measurement of recovery.

3. SOURCES OF HUMAN AND ENVIRONMENTAL EXPOSURE; ENVIRONMENTAL LEVELS

3.1 Industrial Production

Permethrin was first marketed in 1977. Worldwide production figures (1979-1982) are shown in Table 4.

Table 4. World-wide production of permethrin

Year	Production (tonnes)	Reference
1979	800	Wood Mackenzie (1980)
1980	860	Wood Mackenzie (1981)
1981	660 - 700	Wood Mackenzie (1982, 1983)
1982	650	Wood Mackenzie (1983)
1983	600	Wood Mackenzie (1984)
1984	335	Battelle (1986)

3.2 Use Pattern

Permethrin is a photostable synthetic pyrethroid. It possesses a high level of activity against Leptidoptera and is also effective against Hemiptera, Diptera, and Coleoptera. It is a stomach and contact insectide, but it has very little fumigant activity. Permethrin is not plant systemic. It is fast acting and effective against all growth stages, particularly larvae. Permethrin also has significant repellent action. It is effective against insects at low rates of application and is sufficiently photostable to be of wide-ranging practical use in agri-culture.

Permethrin is mostly used on cotton plants (61% of consumption). The major consumer countries in 1980 were the USA (263 tonnes), Brazil (38 tonnes), Mexico (36 tonnes), and Central America (27 tonnes) (Battelle, 1982).

Other crops to which permethrin is applied are corn, soybean, coffee, tobacco, oil seed rape, wheat, barley, alfalfa, vegetables, and fruits. In addition to its pre-harvest usage, permethrin has a potential application in the protection of stored grain. For example, permethrin has been applied to sorghum or wheat in large scale trials in Australia (FAO/WHO, 1981b, 1982b).

Permethrin is also used for the control of insects in household and animal facilities (Battelle, 1982) or in forest pest control, as a fog in mushroom houses, and as a wood preservative. Other applications are in public health, particularly for insect control in aircraft, treatment of mosquito nets, and human lice control.

It is formulated in emulsifiable concentrates (1.25-50%), ultra-low-volume formulations (5%), wettable powders (25%), and fogging formulations (2-5%) (FAO/WHO, 1980b). Permethrin is normally effective at 50 g ai/ha on leaf brassicae, whereas 100 g ai/ha is often needed under more severe conditions in the Americas, Africa, and South-East Asia. The concentration in most working dilutions is 0.04-0.08% (w/v).

3.3 Residues in Food and Other Products

As might be expected for a compound which is non-systemic and also fairly stable on leaf surfaces, the amount of residue found on different parts of crops depends largely on the direct exposure at the time of application. This is particularly marked with leafy vegetables such as lettuce and cabbage where residue levels on wrapper leaves are usually many times (e.g., 10-100) higher than those on central heads (as trimmed for commercial distribution). Similarly, residues on fruit such as lemons, citrus, and kiwi fruits are almost entirely confined to the peel or similar outer protective surfaces. This is illustrated by the 1979 Joint FAO/WHO Meeting on Pesticide Residue (JMPR) evaluation, which contains findings from the examinations of samples of cabbage, lettuce, oranges, melons, and kiwi fruit (FAO/WHO, 1980b).

Residue levels in cotton seeds are influenced by the degree of boll ripening/opening at the time of last spraying. Levels in root and tuber vegetables are usually less than 0.05 mg/kg (FAO/WHO, 1980b).

Ground and aerial applications have been found to yield similar residue levels in a wide range of vegetable and field crops. Similarly, there were no major differences in residue levels in greenhouse curcurbitae and solanaceae following spray and fogging applications at effective rates under similar conditions (FAO/WHO, 1980b).

Supervised trials and residue analyses have been performed on a variety of crops such as field crops, foliar and root vegetables, trees, soft fruits, and fruiting vegetables. Comprehensive summaries of reports (more than 5000 individual residue results on approximately 60 crops from 17 countries) were described in the evaluation reports of the JMPR, (FAO/WHO 1980b, 1981b, 1982b, 1983b, 1984b, 1985b, 1986b). A comprehensive list of maximum residue limits for a large number of commodities resulted from these evaluations (FAO/WHO 1986c).

The rate of decline of residue levels in various crops is fairly slow, half-life periods ranging from about 1 to 3 weeks depending on the crop. However, there is no obvious build-up of residues following repeated application within the rates and frequencies that are needed to obtain good insect control (FAO/WHO, 1980b).

Residues were measured in cotton seeds in supervised trials during 1975-1977 in the USA. When emulsifiable concentrate formulations (25-40%) of permethrin were applied to fields at rates of 110 or 450 g ai/ha (3 to 16 times, until 0 to 76 days before harvest), the average residue level in cotton seeds was 0.03-0.08 mg/kg, the highest values ranging from 0.03 to 0.27 mg/kg in 27 samples (FAO/WHO, 1980b).

Similar results were obtained when sweet corn was treated 6-13 times with 25% emulsifiable concentrate at a rate of 280-450 g ai/ha. The residue levels at 0-4 days after the last application were <0.01-0.12 mg/kg (Ussary, 1978, 1979).

Wheat grains treated with permethrin at a rate of 0.5-5.0 mg/kg revealed a residue level of 0.36-4.5 mg/kg after 9 months of storage (Halls, 1981). When wheat containing a residue level of 1.09 mg/kg was subjected to milling and baking processes, the level of the permethrin residue declined to 0.12 mg/kg in white bread (Halls & Periam, 1980).

Groups of three cows were fed *cis/trans*(40/60)-permethrin at rates of 0.2, 1.0, 10, 50, or 150 mg/kg diet for 28-31 days. Mean plateau levels in whole milk were <0.01 μg/g and 0.3 μg/g at dietary levels of 0.2 mg/kg and 150 mg/kg, respectively. These levels, however, declined rapidly to <0.01 μg/g within 5 days after permethrin administration ceased. Residue levels of <0.01-0.04 μg/g fat and 2.8-6.2 μg/g fat were found in the perirenal fat of cows that were given permethrin at dietary levels of 0.2 mg/kg and 150 mg/kg, respectively (Edwards & Iswaran, 1977; Swaine & Sapiets, 1981a, 1981b).

In studies by Ussary & Braithwaite (1980), cows were given six whole-body sprays of permethrin at a rate of 1.0 g ai/cow with an interval of 14 days between each spray. They were allowed free access to a self-oiler containing a solution of 0.03 g ai/litre (ensuring at least two applications per day for a period of 10 weeks). The cows were housed in premises that were sprayed at a rate of 0.06 g ai/m^2, six sprays taking place with a 14-day interval between sprays (the cows had free access to the premises during spraying). This degree of exposure is at the highest end of the range that is likely to occur in normal husbandry practice. When cows were slaughtered five days after the sixth application, the permethrin levels in muscle, liver, and kidney were low (<0.01 mg/kg tissue). The highest residue levels detected were 0.10 mg/kg and 0.04 mg/kg in the intestinal and subcutaneous fat, respectively.

Lactating cows (three/group) fed permethrin at dose levels of 0, 0.2, 1.0, 10, or 50 mg/kg diet for 28 days showed no mortality, and growth and milk production were normal. Permethrin residues were observed in the milk within 3 days at the two highest dietary levels; levels appeared to reach a plateau rapidly and not to increase with time. Analysis of individual cis and trans isomers showed that the ratio of permethrin isomers in milk appeared to change during the course of the study with the cis isomer predominating. Permethrin residues were not found in the tissues of animals that received doses of 1 mg/kg or less. At dose levels of 10 or 50 mg/kg, residues were detected in the tissues, predominantly in the fat. Low levels were also present in the muscle and kidney at the highest dose level. Permethrin did not appear to accumulate in the fat but to reach a plateau rapidly (Edwards & Iswaran, 1977).

3.4 Residues in the Environment

Data on precise levels of permethrin residues in the air, water, or soil are not available. However, an assessment of the environmental residues resulting from permethrin application has been made in some studies.

Permethrin deposits and airborne concentrations have been measured downwind from a single swath application using a back-pack mist blower. Samples from Kromekote cards (to assess droplet density and size distribution), glass plates, water surface, bronze rods, and air samplers were collected, cleaned up, and analysed by HPLC (Sundaram et al., 1987). Permethrin deposits on all static collectors were greatest within 30 m of the spray swath. Beyond 30 m downwind, the amounts of the insecticide trapped by various collectors were extremely low and were barely detectable.

Lindquist et al. (1987) measured permethrin concentrations in greenhouse air and deposition on glass plates following application by several different methods. Highest airborne residues were found after thermal pulse-jet applications and lowest after hydraulic sprayings. Most airborne residues were detected within 4 h of application. Surface residues were highest after hydraulic and mechanical aerosol applications. Thermal pulse-jet applications resulted in low surface residues.

Agnihotri et al. (1986) evaluated the persistence of permethrin in water and sediment contained in open trenches (3 m x 1 m x 30 cm) lined with alkathene sheet. Insecticide emulsion was sprayed on the surface of water at the normal recommended dosage and at twice this value. The dissipation of the insecticide from the water was rapid, about 87-90% of the pesticide being lost within 24 h at both rates of application. However, residues were found to be absorbed by the sediment and these persisted even beyond 30 days. In soil, persistence was moderate, lasting for around 30 days.

4. ENVIRONMENTAL TRANSPORT, DISTRIBUTION, AND TRANSFORMATION

The degradation pathways of permethrin by ultraviolet light, in soils, and in plants are summarized in Fig. 2.

4.1 Transport and Distribution between Media

In laboratory studies, permethrin in water was rapidly adsorbed onto lake sediments or soil columns and was not desorbed or eluted easily from them. However in forest spray trials, permethrin residues were not only dissipated from water streams very rapidly but also did not accumulate much in the bottom sediment. This was explained by the fact that the low density of permethrin and its insolubility in water prevented it from reaching bottom sediments. Residues in forest litter and exposed soils were more stable. Low levels of degradation products can be translocated from soils to plants.

When a 640-ha forest block in northern Ontario, Canada, was sprayed once with permethrin at 17.5 g ai/ha, residues in water persisted for less than 96 h and attained peak concentrations of 147.0 μg/litre in ponds and 2.5 μg/litre in streams after one hour. Accumulation and persistence of the pesticide in bottom sediment were negligible. Residue levels in the treated streams ranged from 0.05 to 0.89 μg/litre and persisted for a maximum of 96 h, but in another case, residues fell to a non-detectable level (less than 0.05 μg/l) after 6-24 h. Permethrin residues appeared 2.1 km downstream from the treatment block 6 h after spraying. The level reached a peak of 0.18 μg/litre at 12 h and did not persist beyond 96 h. Accumulation of the insecticide in pond sediment was minimal (5-8 μg/kg) and persisted for less than 7 days. No permethrin residue was found in stream sediments. The sprayed permethrin formulation had a density (0.88 g/ml) less than that of water and was practically insoluble in water. It therefore formed a surface film when brought into contact with stagnant or slowly moving water. This significantly reduced the likelihood of the insecticide reaching the bottom sediment or exposing fish in the treated ponds and streams. Insecticide residues in foliage, soil, and litter were more stable than in water and remained at detectable concentrations to the end of the 58-day sampling period. Deciduous and coniferous foliage contained permethrin residues ranging from 0.02 to 0.78 mg/kg and retained concentrations of 0.02-0.05 mg/kg for at least 57 days. Forest litter within the treatment block showed a residue level of 0.07 mg/kg 58 days after the pesticide application. The permethrin residue levels in exposed soil in the treatment block were fairly constant (0.04-0.07mg/kg) for up to 58 days (Kingsbury & Kreutzweiser, 1980a).

In another field test where permethrin was sprayed (17.5 g ai/ha) twice at intervals of 9 or 10 days in two forest blocks in Quebec, Canada, the stagnant water in the sprayed region contained permethrin levels of no more than 0.62 μg/litre and 0.84 μg/litre after the initial and second applications, respectively. Samples from the streams

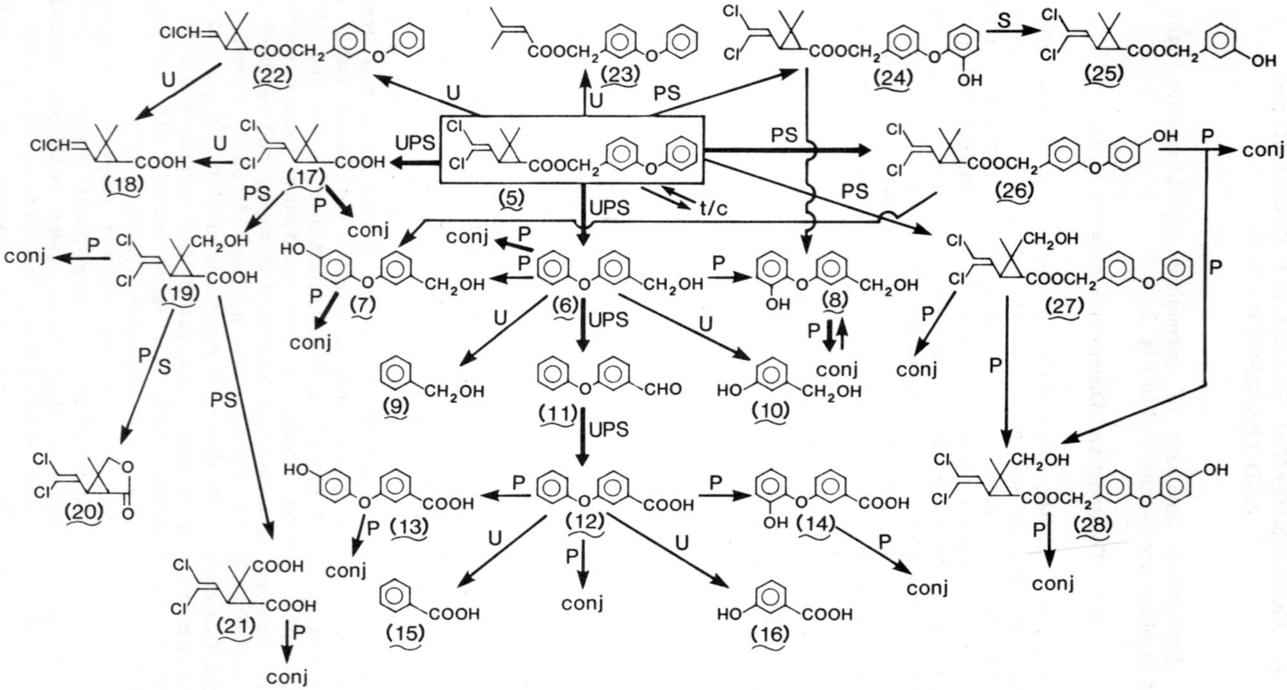

Fig. 2. Degradation pathways of permethrin in plants and soils, and by UV light
U = UV light; P = plant (conj = sugar conjugate); S = soil.

showed residue levels ranging from 0.05 to 1.84 μg/litre. Permethrin concentrations in the water persisted at mean levels of 0.15 μg/litre for 96 h and 0.03 μg/litre for 48 h after the first and second applications, respectively (detection limit: 0.01 μg/litre). Sediments collected from a pond and streams, contained 30-95 μg permethrin/kg. Accumulation of residual permethrin in stream sediment 4.5 km downstream from the treatment block was minimal. Permethrin residue levels in forest litter increased substantially following the second application. Mean concentrations ranged from 0.01 mg/kg to 0.053 mg/kg but fell to non-detectable levels within 59 days (Kreutzweiser, 1982).

In a laboratory adsorption-desorption study, more than 95% of permethrin in aqueous solutions (6-42 μg/litre) was rapidly adsorbed onto lake sediment, and the adsorbed insecticide was not easily desorbed from the sediment by several water rinses. A high distribution coefficient (i.e., g adsorbed per g sediment divided by g per ml of solution) of 389 ml/g was obtained from the adsorption isotherm. Permethrin in aqueous solution applied to the surface of a sediment column did not penetrate through more than 2 cm of the sediment (Sharom & Solomon, 1981).

In a laboratory soil-leaching experiment, ^{14}C-labelled (+)-*cis* or (+)-*trans*-permethrin was incubated with two types of soils (light clay soil of Kodaira and sandy clay loam soil of Azuchi) for 0 day or 21 days, then these permethrin-soil mixtures were applied to the top of a soil column and eluted with water. When a mixture with no pre-incubation was applied to the column, only 1.0 to 3.4% of the radiocarbon was found in lower layer and no radiocarbon was eluted. However, the degradation products from the pre-incubated samples were eluted with water to a slight extent (see section 4.4) (Kaneko et al., 1978).

Similar results were obtained by Kaufman et al. (1981) in soil mobility studies using soil TLC methods.

The uptake of permethrin and its degradation products by plants from soil was studied by Leahey & Carpenter (1980). Sandy loam soil was treated separately with [^{14}C-cyclopropyl]- and [^{14}C-phenyl]-permethrin at a spray application rate of 2 kg/ha. The top 8 cm of the treated soil was thoroughly mixed, and sugar beet, wheat, lettuce, and cotton seeds were sown at intervals of 30, 60, and 120 days after treatment. Low radioactive residues (up to 0.86 mg/kg) were detected in mature plants, but the residues were higher in crops grown in soil treated with [^{14}C-cyclopropyl]-permethrin. It appeared that certain carboxylic acid metabolites formed in the soil were subsequently taken up by the plants. However, under field conditions, no residues of permethrin or its metabolites were detected in crops sown 60 days or more after soil treatment (Swaine et al., 1978).

4.2 Photodecomposition

Appraisal

Photochemical studies of permethrin in thin films and in solution have shown it to be much more stable to light (10-100 times) than synthetic pyrethroids developed earlier. In solution, photoisomerization at the 1,3-bond of the cyclopropane ring and ester cleavage were shown to be the major reactions.

In a thin film on plywood, permethrin remained insecticidally active after 26 days, compared with 4-8 days and <2 days for phenothrin and resmethrin, respectively. When exposed to daylight as a thin film (0.2 mg/cm^2) indoors near a window, phenothrin photodecomposed with a half-life of about 6 days, whereas 60% of applied permethrin remained undecomposed after 20 days. Thus, replacement of the isobutenyl group with the dichlorovinyl substituent significantly enhanced the photostability of permethrin. Permethrin was reported to be 10-100 times more photostable than other pyrethroids synthesized earlier (Elliott et al, 1973).

The photolysis of [1RS,*trans*]- or [1RS,*cis*]-permethrin (5)[a] has been examined using materials labelled with ^{14}C at the carboxy (acid) or benzyl (alcohol) group (Fig. 2). On irradiation with ultraviolet light (peak wavelength: 290-320 nm), both permethrin isomers decomposed slightly faster in hexane than in methanol. In both solvents, the cis isomer photodecomposed about 1.6 times faster ($T_{\frac{1}{2}}$ = 43-58 min) than the trans isomer. The photodecomposition reaction involved extensive isomerization of the cyclopropane ring, i.e. interconversion of the trans and cis isomers. This probably occurred via a triplet energy state forming the diradical intermediate through Cl-C3 bond fission, since the reaction was efficiently quenched by 1,3-cyclohexadiene. The isomerization reaction reached a state of equilibrium after 1-4 h of irradiation and the more thermodynamically stable trans isomer constituted 65-70% of the isomer mixture. Apart from the isomerization reaction, ester cleavage was the major photolytic reaction. As the result of ester cleavage and other photolytic reactions, products formed from permethrin also included smaller or trace amounts of monochloro-permethrin (22) (from reductive dechlorination), 3-phenoxybenzaldehyde (PBald) (11), 3-phenoxybenzoic acid (PBacid) (12), 3-phenoxybenzyl-3,3-dimethylacrylate (23) (from diradical intermediate), and benzyl alcohols (9,10), as well as their corresponding acids (15,16). In addition, large amounts of unidentified polar products were detected, especially in water. Permethrin and monochloro-permethrin (0.1-0.5 g) did not undergo photo-oxidation or other reactions within 7 days in oxygenated methanol solution using Rose Bengal as a sensitizer. Thus the chlorine atoms at the vinyl position had a pronounced effect

---

a Numbers in parentheses refer to the corresponding numbers in Fig.2

in protecting this substituent from oxidation or epoxidation, as compared with the isobutenyl in chrysanthemate (Holmstead et. al., 1978).

Holmstead et al. (1978) also investigated the photodegradation of permethrin on a soil surface. The degradation on soil was similar to the degradation pathways established in solution, but the rate of degradation was slower and photo-isomerisation less important. Exposure of the permethrin isomers on Dunkirk silt loam soil for 48 h resulted in about a 55% loss of permethrin under sunlight and about a 35% loss in the dark. The amount of unextractable material was about 6% in the dark and about 18% in the light. On soil, permethrin did not undergo extensive isomerization of the cyclopropane ring as it did in solution. There was little difference in the amount of free acid detected in the dark or in light, and 3-phenoxybenzyl alcohol (PBalc) (6) (approximately 5%) was the major cleavage product of the alcohol moiety. Other products detected in trace amounts were essentially similar to those present in solutions that had undergone photolysis.

4.3 Degradation in Plants

Appraisal

Thorough investigations of the fate of permethrin in plants have been performed using bean plants and cotton plants. No significant differences in the types of metabolic pathways were detected for the two plant species. Very little translocation of permethrin or its metabolites was observed following either topical application or stem injection of permethrin to plants. Photochemical reactions played an important role in the fate of permethrin applied to the surface of plants. A major degradation pathway in plants was ester cleavage, followed by rapid conjugation with sugars of the Cl_2CA and PBalc thus formed.

The metabolism of the [1R,trans] and [1R,cis] isomers of ^{14}C-permethrin, labelled separately in the dichlorovinyl and benzyl carbon atoms, in snap bean seedlings has been studied in the greenhouse. Whole-body autoradiography of the plants showed that little translocation of radiolabelled permethrin or its metabolites had occurred. The amounts of radiocarbon remaining after 14 days were 13-17% of the dose in the surface wash, 46-58% in the methanol extract, and 8-14% unextracted in the plant residues. Some interconversion of the trans and cis isomers occurred and the cis isomer was slightly more persistent than the trans isomer. The initial half-lives of the cis and trans isomers of permethrin in the seedlings were 9 and 7 days, respectively. A large number of metabolites were detected in the plant extracts, the major ones from the alcohol moiety being PBalc (6) and its corresponding 2′- (8) or 4′-hydroxy (7) derivatives, which occurred mainly as glucoside conjugates (Fig. 1). There were seven or eight additional minor unidentified products. The cis and trans isomers of 3-(2,2-dichlorovinyl)-2,2-dimethylcyclopropanecarboxyclic acid (Cl_2CA) (17) were the major metabolites from the acid moiety and occurred mainly as conjugated forms. In addition, trace amounts of the 2′- (24) or 4′-hydroxy (26) derivatives of permethrin were also detected. From the hydrolysis experiments using β-glucosidase, it was inferred that the sugar concerned was glucose, but no detailed evidence of the identity was obtained (Ohkawa et al., 1977).

In a separate study, Gaughan & Casida (1978) examined the metabolism of the [1RS,trans] and [1RS,cis] isomers of permethrin in snap beans in the glasshouse and in cotton both in the glasshouse and outdoors. Individual leaves of snap beans and cotton plants were treated with 1 μg of *cis*- or *trans*-^{14}C-permethrin labelled either at the carboxy or methylene carbon. Under field conditions, about 30% of the radiolabel was lost from cotton plants within one week after application and some trans/cis isomerization at the cyclopropane ring took place by photodecomposition. *trans*-Permethrin was metabolized more rapidly than the cis isomer. The major degradation pathway was again hydrolysis, followed by rapid conjugation of Cl_2CA (17) and PBalc (6) with sugars. There were at least two types of conjugates; the minor one was a glycoside readily cleaved by β-glucosidase and the major one was a conjugate which was resistant to β-glucosidase but was readily cleaved by cellulase. Other products identified included the hydroxylated compounds reported by Ohkawa et al. (1977) in their study of beans treated with permethrin. In addition, hydroxylation at either of the two methyl groups in the acid moiety (27) with subsequent conjugation occurred to a greater extent with the more stable cis isomer. Similar metabolites to those formed under field conditions were detected in bean and cotton plants under glasshouse conditions.

Roberts & Wright (1981) studied the conjugation of ^{14}C-PBalc in cotton plants using abscised leaves to obtain more information on the nature of the conjugates produced. The alcohol was rapidly converted to glucosyl 3-phenoxybenzyl ether and subsequently to more polar substances such as disaccharide conjugates with glucose and pentose (probably xylose or arabinose) sugars. The alcohol and its monosaccharide and disaccharide conjugates underwent interconversion in the cotton leaves. The evidence was obtained from experiments with ^{14}C-glucose, which showed the ready exchange of the glucose units of the conjugates with free glucose in the leaves. No larger sugar conjugates of PBalc were detected in plants.

From the above studies, it can be concluded that the types of products formed from permethrin in plants are similar to those formed in mammals, except for the nature of the conjugates (see section 5.1).

4.4 Degradation in Soils

Appraisal

Several studies on the degradation of permethrin in a wide variety of soil types have been carried out. These studies used permethrin labelled with ^{14}C at different positions, so that the fate of virtually all of the significant sub-units of the molecule has been traced. In all soil types *degradation is fairly rapid under aerobic conditions, conversion to $^{14}CO_2$ being the major ultimate fate of the ^{14}C. With all soils and all positions of radiolabelling, the formation of unextractable residues is a major occurrence. Under anaerobic conditions, similar degradation processes seem to occur, but the rate of ultimate conversion to $^{14}CO_2$ is slower than under aerobic conditions.*

Kaufman et al. (1977) studied the degradation of cis and trans isomers of permethrin in five soils under aerobic, anaerobic, and sterilized conditions. Soils were treated with ^{14}C-permethrin labelled separately in the carboxy and methylene groups at a dose rate of 224 g/ha and stored under aerobic conditions at 25°C. Degradation of permethrin was rapid in four of five soils, with the trans isomer decomposing more rapidly than the cis isomer. The initial half-lives were less than 28 days in all but one soil. Rapid evolution of $^{14}CO_2$ was observed. In Hagerstown silty clay loam soil, 62% of methylene- and 52% of carboxy-labelled permethrin were converted to $^{14}CO_2$ in 27 days. Only 15% (methylene-labelled) to 19% (carboxy-labelled) of the applied radiolabel was extractable with methanol, 25-27% remaining unextracted and associated with soil organic matter. Microbial metabolism was involved in permethrin degradation and the major route was hydrolysis of the ester linkage to form PBalc and Cl_2CA, the former product being subsequently oxidized to PBacid. In contrast, less than 0.3% of $^{14}CO_2$ was evolved from soils treated with sodium azide (an inhibitor of microbial growth) or when the soil was incubated under waterlogged anaerobic conditions.

Kaneko et al. (1978) reported the degradation in two Japanese soils of ^{14}C-permethrin labelled separately in the dichlorovinyl and methylene groups. The initial half-lives of the trans and cis isomers were 6-9 days and 12 days, respectively, in soils treated at a rate of 1 mg/kg and stored at 25°C under aerobic upland conditions. $^{14}CO_2$ was evolved at rates similar to those observed by Kaufman et al. (1981). As one of the ^{14}C-preparations was different in labelled position from those used in the earlier work, the evolution of $^{14}CO_2$ was the evidence for extensive degradation of the cyclopropyl moiety after hydrolysis in the soils. In addition to the hydrolysis products, several oxidation products were identified, including 3-(2,2-dichlorovinyl)-2-methyl-2-hydroxymethyl-cyclopropanecarboxylic acid (19) and 3-(4-hydroxyphenoxy)benzyl-3-(2,2-dichlorovinyl)-2,2-dimethylcyclopropane-carboxylate (26).

The degradation of permethrin was studied in a flooded Memphis silt loam soil incubated at 25°C, [^{14}C-carbonyl]-*cis*-, [^{14}C-carbonyl]-*trans*-, and [methylene-^{14}C]-*cis*-permethrin being added to the soil at rates of 0.1 and 1.0 mg/kg. The soils were analyzed after 0, 4, 8, 16, 32, and 64 days to determine the distribution of ^{14}C in CO_2, solvent-extractable compounds, water-soluble polar compounds, and soil-bounds residues. Thin-layer chromatographic analysis of the organic solvent extracts showed that *trans*-permethrin was more rapidly degraded than the cis isomer. After 64 days, the amounts of ^{14}C-*trans*-permethrin remaining were 34.2% (at 0.1 mg/kg) and 30.3% (at 1.0 mg/kg) of the applied ^{14}C, and those of ^{14}C-*cis*-permethrin were 73.4% (at 0.1 mg/kg) and 69.8% (at 1.0 mg/kg). Two metabolites, 3-(2,2-dichloro-vinyl)-2,2-dimethylcyclopropanecarboxylic acid (17) and PBalc (6), resulting from permethrin hydrolysis were identified. Other metabolites were PBacid (12) and PBald (11). Fragmentation of (17) and (12) to CO_2 was not extensive, and cumulative $^{14}CO_2$ recoveries were less than 3.5% for all treatments during the 64-day incubation period. The metabolism of *trans*-permethrin resulted in the accumulation of polar compounds in the water. Soil-bound residues gradually increased with time and accounted for 3.3-11.4% of the ^{14}C activity after 64 days. The largest percentage of soil-bound ^{14}C residue was in the fulvic acid fraction (Jordan & Kaufman, 1986).

When ^{14}C-permethrin preincubated with soil for 21 days was applied on top of a soil column and eluted with water, 7.9-17.2% of the applied radiocarbon was recovered in the lower layers of the column and 0.3-2.6% was found in effluents (Kaneko et al., 1978). Only degradation products of permethrin, such as PBacid (12) and 3-(4-hydroxyphenoxy)-benzyl-3-(2,2-dichlorovinyl)-2,2-dimethylcyclopropanecarboxylate (26) were identified in the effluent. Permethrin was not present in the effluent (see section 4.1).

The persistence of permethrin in soil was studied in aqueous suspensions of soil spiked with permethrin at a rate of 17.8 mg/kg under a range of redox potential (-150, +50, +250, and +450 mV) and at pH 5.5, 7.0, and 8.0. The results of this study indicated that both the pH and redox potential significantly influence the degradation of permethrin. After 25 days, permethrin disappeared almost completely under well oxidized (+450 mV) conditions at all three pH levels. Under reduced conditions (-150 mV), only about 40% of the applied permethrin was degraded. The rate of degradation of permethrin was moderate at weakly oxidized (+250 mV) and moderately reduced (+50 mV) conditions at pH 8. Thus, permethrin was lost more rapidly under oxidizing conditions, and increasing the pH enhanced this loss under moderately reduced and weakly oxidized conditions (Gambrell et al., 1981).

Jordan et al. (1982) investigated the effect of temperature on the degradation of permethrin in soil. Dubbs fine sandy loam soil was treated with [^{14}C-carbonyl]-*cis*, *trans*-permethrin at a rate of 1 mg/kg and incubated at 10, 25, and 40°C for up to 64 days. The half-lives of disappearance for *trans* and *cis* isomers were 14 and 55 days at 10°C, 5 and 12 days at 25°C, and 4 and 27 days at 40°C, respectively. The most rapid rate of degradation of permethrin occurred at 25°C, permethrin being converted to Cl_2CA (17) and ultimately to $^{14}CO_2$. At 40°C rapid degradation of permethrin to Cl_2CA also occurred, but further degradation of Cl_2CA to $^{14}CO_2$ was reduced. The amount of $^{14}CO_2$ evolved after 64 days was 56% at 25°C, compared with 29% at 10°C and 24% at 40°C.

Lord et al. (1982) investigated the factors affecting the persistence of permethrin in three loam soils under laboratory conditions.

The degradation of *trans*-permethrin (4 mg/kg) at 30°C was similar at three moisture contents ranging from 40 to 80% of water-holding capacity, but more rapid degradation occurred in an aqueous soil suspension system probably due to better distribution of the insecticide. Four repeated applications of permethrin (4 mg/kg) at 20-day intervals, or addition of nutrients including sucrose (1 mg/kg), powdered cellulose (100 mg/kg), and NH_4Cl (80 mg/kg) plus K_2HPO_4 (260 mg/kg) to soils caused no drastic changes in the rate of degradation of permethrin.

The influence of organic materials on the degradation of permethrin in soil was also studied by Doyle et al. (1981). [^{14}C-carbonyl]-*cis*-permethrin was added to silty loam soil which had been pretreated with sewage sludge or dairy manure at rates of 0, 50, or 100 tonnes/ha, and total CO_2 and $^{14}CO_2$ evolution were monitored regularly throughout a 60-day incubation period at 25°C. The incorporation of sewage or dairy manure at the rate of 50 and 100 tonnes/ha increased permethrin breakdown by 87% and 149% (sewage), or 64% and 134% (dairy manure) based on the values measured in unamended soil, respectively. In the waste-amended soils, a lag period of 28-38 days during which time virtually no $^{14}CO_2$ was evolved, was followed by a rapid evolution of $^{14}CO_2$ before the rate became stabilized. The highest rates (0.21-0.22% per day) were observed in soils amended with either dairy manure or sewage sludge at 100 tonnes/ha. The rate of $^{14}CO_2$ formation correlated directly with the total microbial activity, as measured by total CO_2 production.

In studies by Williams & Brown (1979), the persistence of permethrin in six soils was compared with that of fenvalerate under laboratory conditions. The soils were treated with one of the insecticides at 1 mg/kg and incubated under aerobic conditions for 16 weeks at a temperature alternating between 20°C for 15 h and 10°C for 9 h to simulate the actual field conditions. With the exception of organic soil from Cloverdale, degradation of permethrin was rapid in all soils, with half-lives of 3 weeks or less. Under identical conditions, the half life for fenvalerate was about 7 weeks. Again, *trans*-permethrin was lost more rapidly than the cis isomer, and there was very little loss of either insecticide in the sterilized soils. With Cloverdale organic soil, a greater degree of adsorption onto the soil organic fraction might have contributed to the slower degradation rate.

When soil was treated with [^{14}C-cyclopropyl]-permethrin, sugar beet grown on the treated soil was found to contain radiolabelled conjugates of Cl_2CA and 3-(2,2-dichlorovinyl)-2-methylcyclopropane-1,2-dicarboxylic acid (21) (Leahey & Carpenter, 1980). It was possible that both carboxylic acids were formed in the soil and were subsequently taken up by the plants (see section 4.1).

5. KINETICS AND METABOLISM

5.1 Metabolism in Mammals

Appraisal

The metabolic pathways of permethrin in mammals are summarized in Fig. 3.

The metabolism of permethrin has been studied in great detail in various species of mammals, using a variety of radiolabelled isomers. Permethrin administered to mammals was rapidly metabolized and almost completely eliminated from the body within a short period of time. The trans isomer of permethrin was eliminated more rapidly that the cis isomer. Radiocarbon from trans-permethrin was excreted mostly in urine, whereas that from the cis isomer was eliminated both in urine and faeces to a similar extent. Expiration as CO_2 contributed little to its elimination in mammals. Major routes of metabolism for both trans and cis isomers were ester cleavage and oxidation of the 4′-position of the terminal aromatic ring. A less important reaction in mammals was hydroxylation of the geminal dimethyl group of the cyclopropane ring. Major metabolites thus formed were Cl_2CA in free and glucuronide form, sulfate conjugate of 4′-hydroxy-3-phenoxybenzoic acid, PBacid in free and conjugate form, and hydroxymethyl-Cl_2CA as a glucuronide conjugate. This latter compound was also isolated as a lactone where the hydroxymethyl group and the carboxy group had a cis configuration.

5.1.1 Mouse

In studies by Shah et al. (1981), ^{14}C-*cis*-permethrin was applied to the clipped skin of mice at a level of 1 mg/kg body weight in 0.1 ml of acetone. The mice were restrained until the solvent had evaporated and then placed in mouse metabolism cages. They were sacrificed at 1, 5, 15, 50, 480, and 2880 min after treatment and examined for absorption, distribution, and excretion of the insecticide. About 40% of the applied permethrin had moved from the site of application within 5 min and appeared to move rapidly to other parts of the body.

5.1.2 Rat

When a preparation of [1RS,*trans*]- or [1RS,*cis*]-permethrin (^{14}C-labelled in the alcohol or acid moiety) was administered orally to male rats at levels of 1.6-4.8 mg/kg, the compounds were rapidly metabolized and labels in the acid and alcohol fragments were almost completely eliminated from the body within a few days. The radiocarbon (alcohol or acid label) from the cis isomer was eliminated in the urine (52-54% of the dose) and the faeces (45-47%), whereas 79-82% of the radiocarbon from the trans isomer appeared in the urine and 16-18% in the faeces

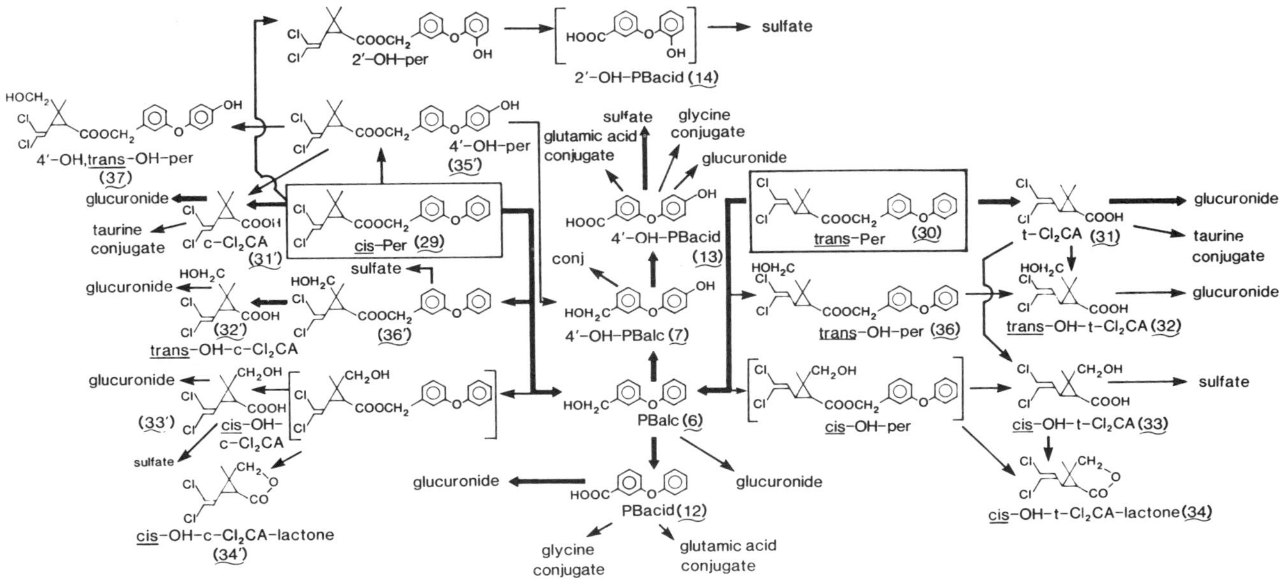

Fig. 3. Metabolic pathways of permethrin in mammals.

within 12 days after administration. The $^{14}CO_2$ contained in the expired air corresponded to less than 0.5% of the dose. The tissue residues were very low, although the cis isomer showed relatively higher residue levels (0.46-0.62 mg/kg tissue) in the fat (Gaughan et al., 1977). The major metabolite from the acid moiety was Cl_2CA (17), which was mostly excreted in the urine, conjugated with glucuronic acid. This accounted for 50-63% of the dose from *trans*-permethrin and 15-22% from *cis*-permethrin. Oxidation at either of the geminal dimethyl groups occurred to the extent of 4.3-10.4% (trans) or 12.2-14.9% (cis), and these oxidised products were eliminated in the urine and faeces as such or as the lactone or glucuronide. The major metabolite from the alcohol moiety was 3-(4′-hydroxyphenoxy)benzoic acid (4′-OH-PBacid) sulfate, accounting for 30.7-42.8% of the dose (trans) and 19.5-29.3% (cis). From *cis*-permethrin, 2′-OH-PBacid sulfate (about 3%) was identified. Another significant metabolite was PBacid, which occurred free and as glucuronide or glycine conjugates, and accounted for 25-31% (trans) and 5.7-10.1% (cis) of the dosed radiocarbon. Except for a trace of PBacid, all the above metabolites from the alcohol moiety were excreted entirely in the urine. However, the faeces of rats dosed with *trans*-permethrin contained 1-2% of the radioactive dose as PBalc. Thus substantial portions of the radioactive metabolites in the recovered excreta were identified. The proposed metabolic pathways for cis- and *trans*-permethrin are shown in Fig. 2. The five principle sites of metabolic attack in both permethrin isomers were ester cleavage, oxidation at the *trans*- and *cis*-methyl of the geminal dimethyl group of the acid moiety, and oxidation at the 2′- and 4′-positions of the phenoxy group. Conjugation of the resultant carboxylic acids, alcohols, and phenols with glucuronic acid, glycine, and sulfuric acid occurred to varying extent. *cis*-Permethrin (29) was more stable than *trans*-permethrin (30), and the cis isomer yielded four faecally excreted ester metabolites that resulted from hydroxylation at the 2′- or 4′-position of the phenoxy group or at the *trans*- or *cis*-methyl group on the cyclopropane ring (e.g., (35′), (36′)). The ester-cleaved metabolites were extensively excreted into the urine whereas the metabolites retaining an ester bond were found only in the faeces. The major metabolite from the acid moiety of both isomers was Cl_2CA (31,31′) in free (1-8%) and glucuronide (14-42%) forms. Other significant metabolites were *trans*-OH-Cl_2CA (32,32′) (1-5%) and *cis*-OH-Cl_2CA (33,33′) in the free (3-5%), lactone (34,34′) (0-4%) and glucuronide (1-2%) forms. On the other hand, the alcohol moiety released after cleavage of the ester bond of both isomers was converted mainly to the sulfate of 3-(4′-hydroxyphenoxy)benzoic acid (4′-OH-PBacid) (13) (29-43% of the dose) and PBacid (12) in the free (1-10%) and glucuronide (7-15%) forms. Other significant metabolites of the alcohol moiety were PBalc (6), PBacid-glycine and the sulfate of 3-(2′-hydroxyphenoxy) benzoic acid (2′-OH-PBacid) (14). [1RS,*trans*]- and [1RS,*cis*]-permethrin showed no significant differences in metabolic fate in the rat from [1R,*trans*]- and [1R,*cis*]-permethrin, respectively (Elliott et al., 1976; Gaughan et al., 1977).

5.1.3 Goat

When ten consecutive oral doses of ^{14}C-*trans*- or ^{14}C-*cis*-permethrin (labelled in the acid or alcohol moieties) at 0.2-0.3 mg/kg body weight/day were given to lactating goats, they excreted 72-79% and 25-36% of the trans and cis isomer doses, respectively, in urine and 12-15% and 52-68%, respectively, in the faeces. The amounts of the radiocarbon appearing in the milk were less than 0.7% with any one of the four ^{14}C-labelled preparations. Concerning the tissue residues 24h after the last dose, detectable levels of radiocarbon were found in most tissues, but none was higher than 0.04 mg/kg for the trans isomer or 0.25 mg/kg for the cis isomer (Hunt & Gilbert, 1977).

The permethrin metabolites in goats were formed through cleavage of the ester linkage, hydroxylation at the *cis*- or *trans*-methyl of the geminal dimethyl group, and hydroxylation at the 4'-position of the phenoxybenzyl moiety. Some of these metabolic products were further oxidized and/or conjugated with glycine, glutamic acid and glucuronic acid. The major compounds found in faeces after dosing with *cis*-permethrin were unmetabolized parent compound, 4'-OH-permethrin (35'), *trans*-OH-permethrin (36'), PBalc, *cis*-OH-*cis*-Cl_2CA-lactone (34') and eight unidentified ester metabolites (Fig. 2). The faeces of goats treated with the trans isomer contained large amounts of the parent compound (41-79% of the faecal ^{14}C) and of PBalc (8-25%) and *cis*-OH-*trans*-Cl_2CA-lactone (34). Also, three unidentified ester metabolites were found (8-23%). On the other hand, major urinary metabolites from the alcohol moiety of both isomers were PBacid-glycine (7-9% of the urinary ^{14}C) and 4'-OH-PBacid-glycine (4-12%). PBalc, PBacid, 4'-OH-PBalc (7), 4'-OH-PBacid, PBacid-glutamic acid and 4'-OH-PBacid-glutamic acid were also identified as minor metabolites. The urine of goats treated with both isomers contained, as major components, Cl_2CA in the free form (2-47% of the urinary ^{14}C) and as a glucuronide (27-71%). Cl_2CA-glucuronide was obtained to a larger extent with the trans isomer than with the cis isomer. Other major metabolites of the cis isomer were *cis*-OH-Cl_2CA (33) (9-11%) and *cis*-OH-*cis*-Cl_2CA-lactone (34) (11-16%). *trans*-OH-Cl_2CA (32,32') was detected as a minor metabolite of both isomers. The milk of goats contained the parent compounds, PBacid-glycine, and 4'-OH-PBacid-glycine. On administration of the cis isomer, a larger amount of the parent compound was excreted in the milk than in the case of the trans isomer. Comparatively, when the trans isomer was administered, PBacid-glycine was detected in the milk to a larger extent than with the cis isomer. Most of the radioactivity in the fat was attributable to the parent compound or ester metabolites such as *trans*-OH-permethrin (36,36') and *trans*-OH-permethrin conjugate (Ivie & Hunt, 1980).

5.1.4 Cow

When four lactating Jersey cows were orally administered ^{14}C-*trans*- or *cis*-permethrin preparations (labelled either in the alcohol or acid moiety; three doses of ≈ 1 mg/kg body weight at 24-h intervals), the radiocarbon was almost completely eliminated in the faeces and urine 12 or 13 days after the initial dose. There was more faecal elimination of the radiocarbon and higher tissue residue levels in the fat with the cis isomer than the trans isomer. The ^{14}C blood level reached a transient peak shortly after each dose and decreased to an insignificant level within 2 to 4 days after the last dose. Higher blood levels were attained with ^{14}C-*trans*-permethrin labelled in the acid moiety than when labelled in the alcohol moiety. This difference arising from labelling positions was not evident with *cis*-permethrin. The radiocarbon excreted in the milk was less than 0.5% of the dose. The lowest ^{14}C level in milk was obtained from ^{14}C-*trans*-permethrin (acid moiety labelling) and the highest with ^{14}C-trans-permethrin (alcohol moiety labelling). With all labelled preparations, however, the radiocarbon levels in milk decreased to <100 μg/litre within 2 to 4 days after treatment ceased. The only radiolabelled compound recovered from milk, in the case of the trans isomer, was unmetabolized permethrin, whereas with the cis isomer 85% of the radiocarbon was as parent compound and 15% as *trans*-OH-*cis*-permethrin (36′). The metabolic reactions of permethrin in cows were similar to those in rats and hens. In cows, the permethrin isomers, their mono- and dihydroxy derivatives, and PBalc, appeared only in the faeces, while the *cis*-OH-Cl_2CA-lactones (34,34′) appeared in both faeces and urine. The remaining metabolites appeared only in the urine. Although a slightly larger portion of *cis*-permethrin than *trans*-permethrin was excreted unchanged, there were similar amounts of ester metabolites with both isomers. These ester metabolites were hydroxylated at the *trans*- or *cis*-methyl positions of the geminal dimethyl group, at the 4′-position of the phenoxybenzyl group, or at both the geminal dimethyl and phenoxy groups. The preferred hydroxylation site with both isomers was the *trans*-methyl group. The major metabolites from the acid moieties of both isomers was the corresponding *cis*-OH-Cl_2CA (33,33′) and its lactone and Cl_2CA-glucuronide, while *trans*-OH-*cis*-Cl_2CA (32′) was also a major metabolite from *cis*-permethrin. On the other hand, the major metabolites from the alcohol moiety of both isomers were PBacid-glycine (3-11% of the dose), PBalc (8-10%), and PBacid-glutamic acid (12-28%) (Gaughan et al., 1978a).

5.1.5 Man

Two human volunteers, who consumed about 2 and 4 mg of permethrin (25:75), respectively, excreted 18-37% and 32-39% of the administered dose, detected as the metabolite Cl_2CA, after acid hydrolysis of their urine collected over 24 h (Cridland & Weatherley, 1977a,b).

5.2 Metabolism in Hens

A mixture (cis:trans = 25:75) of permethrin labelled with ^{14}C in the alcohol moiety was sprayed on 28 hens at doses of 3.77 or 11.94 mg/hen. The hens treated with the low dose showed no detectable levels of radiocarbon in the gizzard, heart, lung, muscle, or egg white 24 h after spraying, but the radiocarbon in the egg yolk reached a maximum level of 0.049 mg/kg 5 days after treatment. The concentration of permethrin residues in the fat reached a peak 7 days after treatment and no significant radioactivity was detectable after 4 weeks. With the high dose, the radiocarbon in the skin had reached 6.69 mg/kg after 3 days. Small quantities of the radiocarbon were found in the egg yolks (0.121 mg/kg) after 5 days and fat (0.110 mg/kg) after 1 day (Hunt et al., 1979).

When White Leghorn hens were treated orally three consecutive days with one of four ^{14}C-*trans*- and *cis*-permethrin isomers labelled in the alcohol or acid moieties at 10 mg/kg body weight, they showed no signs of poisoning. More than 87% of the radiocarbon from the four labelled preparations was found in the excreta 9 days after the initial dose, 0.7-4.7% of the dose was exhaled as $^{14}CO_2$, and 0.12-0.47% and 0.06-0.66% of the radiocarbon was recovered in egg yolk and fat (subcutaneous and visceral fat), respectively. Both the cis isomers labelled in the alcohol and acid moieties showed recoveries 3 to >10 times higher in the fat and egg yolk than those shown by the corresponding trans isomers. The excreta (0-72 h) contained 1.7 times more *cis*-permethrin than *trans*-permethrin. Hydroxylated ester metabolites of *trans*-permethrin were not excreted, but four monohydroxy and dihydroxy esters (i.e. *trans*-OH-permethrin, 4'-OH-permethrin, 4'-OH, *trans*-OH-permethrin (37) and *trans*-OH-permethrin sulfate) of *cis*-permethrin were found. Metabolites from the acid moieties of both isomers were the Cl_2CA isomers in free, glucuronide, and taurine conjugate forms, *trans*-OH-Cl_2CA (32,32'), *cis*-OH-Cl_2CA (33,33'), *cis*-OH-Cl_2CA lactone (34,34'), and *cis*-OH-Cl_2CA sulfate. *trans*-OH-Cl_2CA (32,32') was obtained from the cis isomer to larger extents than from the trans isomer, whereas the amounts of *cis*-OH-Cl_2CA (33,33') were larger with the trans isomer than with the cis isomer. The metabolites from the alcohol moiety included PBalc, PBacid, their 4'-hydroxy-derivatives and the corresponding sulfate, the glucuronide of PBalc, and a variety of unidentified conjugates of 4'-OH-PBalc (7) and 4'-OH-PBacid (13). The taurine conjugate of PBacid was not detected. The metabolites produced in largest amounts were the unidentified conjugates of 4'-OH-PBalc (6-13% of the dose) and 4'-OH-PBacid (2-11%). The yolk of eggs 5 and 6 days after initial dosing contained 4.4 times more *cis*-permethrin than *trans*-permethrin in unchanged form and the same ester metabolites of *cis*-permethrin as those found in the excreta. Other metabolites in the yolk were generally the same as those in the excreta. Overall, *cis*-permethrin appeared at higher levels than *trans*-permethrin in the egg yolk, fatty tissues, and excreta. Radiocarbon from *cis*-permethrin preparations also persisted longer in the blood than that from *trans*-perpermethrin preparations. It probably resulted from more rapid ester cleavage of the trans isomer than the cis isomer, based on the relative amounts of hydrolysis products from the two isomers in hen excreta (Gaughan et al., 1978b).

5.3 Enzymatic Systems for Biotransformation

In studies by Shono et al. (1979), 1 μg each of [1RS,*trans*]-permethrin or [1RS,*cis*]-permethrin was incubated at 37°C for 30 min with 2.2 ml of ≈10% rat and mouse liver microsomes under the following conditions:

- microsomes treated with tetraethyl pyrophosphate (TEPP) (no esterase and oxidase activity),
- normal microsomes (esterase activity),
- TEPP-treated microsomes plus NADPH (oxidase activity),
- normal microsomes plus NADPH (esterase plus oxidase activity).

Each esterase preparation hydrolyzed *trans*-permethrin to a much greater extent than the corresponding cis isomer. In contrast, oxidative metabolism was greater for *cis*-permethrin than for *trans*-permethrin except with the mouse microsomes, where the reactions of both isomers proceeded to a similar extent. Aryl hydroxylation occurred at the 4'- and 6-positions with the mouse enzymes but only at the 4'-position with the rat enzymes. Hydroxylation at the 2'-position was observed only with the *cis*-permethrin and mouse oxidase system. The amount of *trans*-hydroxymethyl ester metabolites exceeded that of the corresponding *cis*-hydroxymethyl compounds except with rat enzymes acting on *trans*-permethrin. In general, oxidative activity with rat microsomes was weaker than that with mouse microsomes. The dihydroxy ester metabolite was evident only with *cis*-permethrin. The *cis*-hydroxymethyl ester derivatives of *trans*-permethrin were further oxidized to the corresponding aldehyde and carboxylic acid by the mouse enzymes. The preferred sites of hydroxylation, based on all identified metabolites in the oxidase and esterase-plus-oxidase systems, were as follows (Shono et al., 1979):

trans-permethrin

mouse:	*cis*-methyl > *trans*-methyl > 4'-carbon = 6-carbon
rat:	4'-carbon = *cis*-methyl > *trans*-methyl

cis-permethrin

mouse:	*trans*-methyl > *cis*-methyl = 4'-carbon > 6-carbon > 2'-carbon
rat:	4'-carbon = *trans*-methyl > *cis*-methyl

When 100 nmol each of [1R,*trans*]-, [1S,*trans*]-, [1RS,*trans*]-, [1R,*cis*]-, [1S,*cis*]-, or [1RS,*cis*]-permethrin were incubated individually with 2.5 ml of mouse liver microsome (1.5-2.0 mg of protein), the trans isomers were much more rapidly hydrolyzed than the corresponding cis isomers. Of the trans isomers, [1S,trans] isomer was hydrolyzed to a greater extent than the other trans isomers. On the other hand, when esterase activity was suppressed, there were no distinct differences in the oxidative metabolic rates between trans and cis isomers (Soderlund & Casida, 1977).

The persistence of isomers of permethrin, cypermethrin, deltamethrin, and fenvalerate in the fat and brain after oral or intraperitoneal administration of these pesticides to rats was compared by

Marei et al. (1982). Residues in fat and brain were much higher and more persistent with *cis*-permethrin than with *trans*-permethrin or the α-cyano-phenoxybenzyl pyrethroids (cypermethrin, fenvalerate, deltamethrin). Brain levels of *trans*-permethrin (but not of *cis*-permethrin) were greatly elevated after pretreatment with pyrethroid esterase and oxidase inhibitors (i.e. tri-*o*-cresyl phosphate, *S,S,S*-tributyl phosphorotrithioate, phenyl saligenin cyclic phosphanate as esterase inhibitors and piperonyl butoxide as oxidase inhibitor).

Pyrethroid carboxyesterase(s) that hydrolyze esters of chrysanthemic acid were purified by Suzuki & Miyamoto (1978) from rat liver microsomes by cholic acid solubilization, ammonium sulfate fractionation, heat treatment, and DEAE-Sephadex A-50 column chromatography. The 45-fold purified enzyme (38% yield) was thought to consist of a single protein with a relative molecular mass of approximate 74 000, a Michaelis constant (Km) of 0.21 mmol/litre for [1R,*trans*]-phenothrin, and an optimum pH of 7-9. It was susceptible to inhibition by organophosphate and carbamate insecticides and insensitive to *p*-chloromercurybenzoic acid and to mercuric and cupric ions. The enzyme seemed to require neither coenzymes nor cofactors and hydrolysed trans isomers of several synthetic pyrethroids (tetramethrin, resmethrin, *trans*- or *cis*-phenothrin and permethrin) well, at more or less similar rates. On the other hand, the cis isomers were hydrolysed at rates one-fifth to one-tenth of those of the trans counterparts. The purified pyrethroid carboxyesterase was apparently identical in nature to malathion carboxyesterase and *p*-nitro phenyl acetate carboxyesterase (Suzuki & Miyamoto, 1978).

6. EFFECTS ON THE ENVIRONMENT

Acute toxicity data of permethrin on aquatic and terrestrial non-target organisms are summarized in Tables 5 and 6, respectively.

6.1 Toxicity to Aquatic Organisms

6.1.1 Aquatic microorganisms

Stratton & Corke (1982) investigated the toxicity of permethrin and ten of its degradation products on the growth, photosynthesis, and acetylene-reducing activity of two species of green algae (*Chlorella pyrenoidosa* and *Scenedesmus quadricaudata*) and three species of cyanobacteria (*Anabaena* spp.). Permethrin itself was relatively non-toxic to photosynthesis (EC_{50} values >100 mg/litre) and to acetylene reduction (EC_{50} values >100 mg/litre). Its degradation products were similarly non-toxic to green algae. However, the cyanobacteria were susceptible to some of the breakdown products of permethrin. Growth was the most sensitive parameter with growth yield showing EC_{50} values of 2.5, 2.2, and 1.4 mg/litre for the cyanobacteria and 2.8 and 4.3 mg/litre for the green algae with PBalc and similar values for three of the five test species with PBald. A complex test system found interactions between the various metabolites and the parent compound which were sometimes additive and sometimes synergistic. The authors concluded that it is difficult to assess the true toxicity of compounds to soil and water microorganisms without considering the breakdown products. The cyanobacteria are significant nitrogen-fixing organisms in wet tropical soils.

6.1.2 Aquatic invertebrates

Non-target invertebrates, except molluscs, are more sensitive to permethrin than fish, as shown in Table 5.

During exposure of permethrin for up to 28 days, the caddisfly (*Brachycentrus americanus*) and the stonefly (*Pteronarcys dorsata*) showed behavioural changes or death at concentrations as low as 0.022 µg/litre (Anderson, 1982).

A 3-h exposure to permethrin, at 50 mg/litre, was not lethal to *Daphnia pulex*. The no-effect levels were 1 µg/litre for racemic, 1R or (+)-trans, and 1R or (+)-cis, and 50 µg/litre for 1S or (-)-trans and 1S or (-)-cis isomers (Miyamoto, 1976).

Zitko et al. (1979) established lethal threshold values for the lobster *Homarus americanus* of 7.00 µg/litre for technical permethrin and 0.40 µg/litre for [1R,*cis*]-permethrin.

Larval oyster and bullfrog (tadpole) are highly tolerant to the insecticide, with LC_{50} values of >1000 and 7000 µg/litre, respectively.

Stratton & Corke (1981) reported that the 48-h LC_{50} of permethrin to juvenile and adult waterfleas *Daphnia magna* was 0.2-0.6 μg/litre. A further series of experiments involved the addition of algae or bacteria to the cultures of daphnids, since feeding of daphnids during these tests had been reported to reduce the toxicity of several chemicals to the animals. With permethrin, however, algae in the test vessel *increased* the lethal effect of the compound. Algae, bacteria, and also inert silica powder adhered to the swimming antennae of the daphnids, causing the daphnids to sink and die on the bottom of the flasks. The effect was greatest with adults; the shed carapaces of juvenile showed the same adhesion of particulates but moulting protected the juveniles to some degree. This raised toxicity was due to a direct effect of the permethrin on the daphnids and not to a tendency for the compound to cause flocculation of the suspended material.

Friesen et al. (1983) tested the toxicity of permethrin to sediment-living nymphs of the mayfly *Hexagenia rigida*. In test vessels containing water without sediment, the 6-h LC_{50} was estimated to lie between 0.58 and 2.06 μg/litre; no nymphs survived exposure to water concentrations of 7.63 μg/litre. In the presence of sediment, lethality was reduced; there was 88% mortality of nymphs exposed to permethrin in water at 7.63 μg/litre after 24-h exposure. Mortality reached 100% only after 7 days exposure with sediment. Maximum concentrations of permethrin in the sediment over the 7 days were estimated to be 50 μg/kg dry weight. The authors also exposed nymphs to sediment previously exposed to permethrin. The initial water concentration was again 7.63 μg/litre, and the sediment was left for 8 days to take up the insecticide before the water was decanted off. Nymphs were introduced along with clean water over the contaminated sediment. There was 100% mortality in the exposed nymphs. Long-term exposure to both water and sediment contaminated with permethrin led to increasing mortality up to 4 weeks; there was little further mortality between 4 and 10 weeks. Lethality reached 100% after exposure to either water or sediment at a simulated application rate of 7.3 g/ha over 10 weeks (95% at 4 weeks), whereas a simulated exposure equivalent to 0.6 g/ha led to 74% mortality after a 10-week exposure of the nymphs in water and 45% after exposure of the nymphs to sediment. The authors comment that it is not yet possible to state a concentration of permethrin in sediment which is sufficiently low to permit successful recolonization of contaminated sediment.

6.1.3 Fish

Permethrin is highly toxic to fish, as shown in Table 5. Preparations using an emulsifiable concentrate of permethrin enhanced its toxicity twofold (Coats & O'Donnell-Jeffery, 1979).

The lethal toxicity of permethrin varied inversely with water temperature, particularly between 10 and 20°C, and with body weight between 1 and 50 g. There was a 10-fold difference between the 96-h LC_{50} values at 10 and 20°C. At 15°C, a large trout (200 g) was considerably more (about 100 times) tolerant than a small fish (1 g) (Kumaraguru & Beamish, 1981).

Toxicity to fish is linked more with the nature of the optical isomers than with that of the stereoisomers; i.e. 1R isomers are more toxic than 1S isomers. Trans and cis isomers are of similar toxicity (Miyamoto, 1976).

Zitko et al. (1979) established lethal threshold values for the Atlantic salmon *Salmo salar* of 8.8 μg/litre for technical permethrin and 1.34 μg/litre for [1R,*cis*]-permethrin.

Hansen et al. (1983) exposed embryos and the hatched fry of sheepshead minnow (*Cyprinodon variegatus*), continuously over 28 days, to concentrations of permethrin of 1.25, 2.5, 5.0, 10, 20, or 40 μg/litre. The survival of embryos was unaffected by any of the test concentrations. Fry were affected by exposure to 20 μg/litre or more but unaffected by 10 μg/litre. The toxicity curve was steep; 99% of fry survived at 10 μg/litre but only 1% at 20 μg/litre. The authors estimated the ratio between the 96-h LC_{50} and the NOEL to be 0.8.

Holdway & Dixon (1988) exposed larval fish (white sucker, *Catastomus commersoni*, and flagfish, *Jordanella floridae*) to permethrin in a single 2-h pulse and examined lethality over the following 96-h. They examined the effect of age, and whether or not the fish were fed, upon the toxic effect of the insecticide. Feeding decreased the toxicity of permethrin to flagfish at 2 and 4 days of age but not at 8 days. Age was the most important factor affecting toxicity. The 96-h LC_{50} (from exposure for 2 h) was 5.55 mg/litre, 7.91 mg/litre, and 0.57 mg/litre for flagfish of age 2, 4, and 8 days, respectively. White suckers were most susceptible to permethrin at 20 days of age, with a 2-h LC_{50} of 10.0 μg/litre. Unfed white suckers at 13 and 20 days of age were highly susceptible to permethrin, with LC_{50} values of 2.0 and 1.0 μg/litre, respectively. The authors pointed out that permethrin is toxic to cladocerans (waterfleas) at levels of 0.5 μg/litre and that fish could suffer both from the direct toxic effect of the insecticide and the added effect experienced during food deprivation.

When used for mosquito control, the safety margins (LC_{50} fish/LC_{50} mosquito larvae) for permethrin and *cis*-permethrin are 2-40 and 25-65, respectively (Mulla et al., 1978a). When intraperitoneally injected into rainbow trout, the *trans*- and *cis*-permethrin isomers were about 110 and 5 times, respectively, more toxic to trout than to mice, (Glickman et al., 1981).

Rainbow trout exposed to sublethal concentrations of permethrin in water (0.09-0.35 μg/litre) or in food (85-350 μg/kg) in 20-40-day experiments showed similar branchial changes, i.e. epithelial separation or necrosis, mucus cell hyperplasia, clubbing of epithelial cells, or hyperplasia and fusion of adjacent secondary lamellae (Kumaraguru et al., 1982).

6.1.4 Field studies and community effects

In studies by Mulla et al. (1975), permethrin was applied to ponds at rates of 56 g/ha and 112 g/ha in field trials. The numbers of *Tanypodinae* (mostly *Pentaneura* and *Tanypus*) and *Chironominae* (mostly

Tanytarsus and *Chironomus*) midge larvae were slightly depressed by the 56 g/ha treatment. Mayfly (mostly *Baetis* sp.) naiads and diving beetle (*Hydrophilidae* and *Dytiscidae*) larvae and adults were also affected. However, *Copepoda* (mostly *Cyclops* and *Diaptomus*) and *Ostracoda* (mostly *Cypricercus* and *Cyprinotus*) were not greatly affected. The effect on these non-target organisms was much greater at the higher dose level of permethrin, except for the ostracods. It was concluded that permethrin affected mayfly naiads severely during the exposure period. Most populations recovered within 2 weeks following exposure.

Mayfly naiads (mostly baetids) were also adversely affected by permethrin at 5.6-28 g/ha and by its cis isomer at 2.8-28 g/ha. There was a slight recovery within 1-3 weeks after treatment (Mulla et al., 1978b).

Permethrin was applied weekly for 6 or 8 successive weeks at the mosquito larvicidal rate of 28 g/ha (and at a rate 5 times higher) to ponds where 20 individuals of mosquito fish or desert pupfish were maintained. The insecticide produced no adverse effects on the two species of fish, and the number of fish in the treated ponds increased markedly during the experiment. At the higher rate, mats of algae were formed, probably as the result of elimination by permethrin of herbivorous arthropods that feed on the algae (Mulla et al., 1981).

Kaushik et al. (1985) investigated the effect of permethrin on the pelagic zooplankton of a 10-ha lake in southern Ontario, Canada. The insecticide was applied to give nominal water concentrations of 0.5, 5.0, or 50 μg/litre in *in situ* aquatic enclosures of 5 x 5 x 5 m. Macrozooplankton (daphnids and copepods) were most susceptible to the insecticide. The numbers, which in untreated enclosures were 100-1000 organisms per litre of water, fell in the days immediately following treatment to 1-10 at 0.5 μg/litre, 0.1-1.0 at 5.0 μg/litre, and 0.01-0.1 organisms per litre at 50 μg/litre of permethrin (nominal). Microzooplankton (mainly rotifers) were unaffected by all doses except the highest. At this dose, numbers fell transitorily to about one tenth of their control levels (about 1000 organisms per litre). In all cases of treatment, rotifer numbers increased between 5- and 10-fold 20 to 100 days after treatment. The authors attributed this rise in numbers to the resistance of the organisms to the insecticide coupled with a reduction in the predator organisms that normally feed on the rotifers. Populations of macrozooplankton had returned to normal within 250 days of treatment (after the winter freeze) even with the highest dose of 50 μg/litre. Recovery was quicker with the lower doses (about 60 days for treatment at 5 μg/litre and 30 days for most species at 0.5 μg/litre). Despite this recovery in overall numbers of zooplankton, there was a decrease in the species diversity of the larger, predator organisms at all treatment levels. The enclosures, of course, prevented immigration from the surrounding areas of water.

Helson et al. (1986) placed two species of aquatic arthropods (the amphipod *Gammarus pseudolimnaeus* and the mosquito *Aedes aegypti*) in open containers of different sizes downwind from the application of permethrin to young spruce trees for control of defoliators. The insecticide was applied to trees 0.75-0.8 m tall in a single swath from a mistblower backpack. Nominal application rates of 36 g ai/ha were used with a swath width of 10 m, and standard and ultra-low volume applications were made. The mortality of *Gammarus* after 48 h averaged 95% (range 76-100%) in the first trial and 85% (range 37-100%) in a duplicate trial in containers 10 m downwind from the spraying. The effect was reduced to 12% and 18% at a distance of 30 m from the spraying and further reduced to an average of 5% 50 m from the spray. Mosquito larvae were examined only in the second trial and showed 76% (37-100%) at 10 m falling to 6% and 2% at 30 and 50 m, respectively, from the spray. Mortality increased over the following 9 days. The authors also determined 48-h LC_{50} values for the two organisms in containers similarly placed in the field. These were 0.37 μg/litre and 0.69 μg/litre for *Gammarus* and mosquito larvae, respectively, while LC_{95} values were 0.61 μg/litre for *Gammarus* and 1.14 μg/litre for mosquito larvae. The authors regarded these data as a "worst case", since sediment in natural water and flowing water in streams could be expected to reduce the toxic effect of the permethrin. They concluded that a 30-m safety zone needs to be left using this application method between a spraying area and natural waters to avoid killing aquatic arthropods.

When permethrin was applied by airplane to the surface of a creek at a nominal rate of 70 g ai/ha, the actual concentration that reached the ground was 13.4 g ai/ha. Dramatic, but short-lived, increases in the drift of aquatic insects (particularly large catches of springtail (*Collembola*), mayfly nymphs (*Ephemeroptera heptageniidea*), water scavenger beetle larvae (*Coleoptera hydrophilidae*), midge larvae and pupae, water boatmen (*Hemiptera corixidae*), predaceous diving beetles (*Coleoptera dytiscidae*), and caddisfly larvae (*Trichoptera*)) occurred after treatment. No effects on populations of organisms that inhabited the bottom layer of the creek were noticeable. The permethrin sprayed had little effect on caged or native fish and no fish mortality was recorded due to the treatment. From these data, it could be inferred that permethrin had no significant impact on the aquatic system (Kingsbury, 1976).

After an aerial application of permethrin at 17.5 g ai/ha, residues attained peak concentrations of 147.0 μg/litre in ponds and 2.5 μg/litre in streams, but accumulations and persistence of the pesticide in bottom sediment were negligible. Noticeable increases in the number of drifting organisms occurred in the treatment block (*Ephemeroptera heptageniidae, Baetidae,* and *Plecoptera* nymphs) and 2.1 km downstream (mayfly and stonefly nymphs) over a 24-h period immediately after the spray. A slight reduction in the bottom fauna also occurred downstream. When exposed in cages in the ponds, yellow perch (*Perca fluvescens*) did not exhibit any adverse effects; little or no accumulated permethrin residues were detectable in the fish following exposure. Observations of the headwater ponds indicated that permethrin application resulted in noticeable levels of distress and mortality to surface and littoral invertebrates and produced a similar impact on benthic organisms (Kingsbury & Kreutzweiser, 1980a).

Table 5. Acute toxicity of permethrin to non-target aquatic organisms

Species	Size	Duration of test	Toxicity[a] (µg/litre)	Formulation[d]	System[e]	Temperature (°C)	pH	Hardness	Reference
A. Freshwater Organisms									
Arthropods									
Crayfish (*Procambarus clarkii*)	0.8 - 1.2 cm, (0.05 g)	96 h	0.39	EC	S	24		100	Jolly et al. (1978)
	2 - 3 cm, (0.5 g)	96 h	0.62	EC	S	24		100	Jolly et al. (1978)
Water flea (*Daphnia pulex*)		3 h	> 50 000	T	S	25			Miyamoto (1976)
		3 h	> 50 000	(+)-trans	S	25			Miyamoto (1976)
		3 h	> 50 000	(+)-cis	S	25			Miyamoto (1976)
		3 h	> 50 000	(-)-trans	S	25			Miyamoto (1976)
		3 h	> 50 000	(-)-cis	S	25			Miyamoto (1976)
Water flea (*Daphnia magna*)	1st instar	48 h	1.26	T	S	18	7.4	42	Mayer & Ellersieck (1986)
Amphipod (*Gammarus pseudolimnaeus*)	immature	96 h	0.17	T	S	17	7.4	42	
Midge (*Chironomus plumosus*)	3rd instar	48 h	0.56	T	S	22	7.4	42	Mayer & Ellersieck (1986)
Caddisfly (*Brachycentrus americanus*)		21 days	0.17	T	F	15	7.6 - 7.8	46 - 48	Anderson (1982)
Fish									
Salmon (*Salmo salar*)	6.2 cm, 5.3 g	96 h	12	T	R	10			McLeese et al. (1980)
Rainbow trout (*Salmo gairdneri*)	1 g	96 h	0.62	T	F	5	7.9 - 8.2	358 - 363	Kumaraguru & Beamish (1981)
	1 g	96 h	0.69	T	F	10	7.9 - 8.2	358 - 363	
	1 g	96 h	3.17	T	F	15	7.9 - 8.2	358 - 363	Kumaraguru & Beamish (1981)
	1 g	96 h	6.43	T	F	20	7.9 - 8.2	358 - 363	
	5 g	96 h	6.43	T	F	15	7.9 - 8.2	358 - 363	Kumaraguru & Beamish (1981)
	20 g	96 h	≈50	T	F	15	7.9 - 8.2	358 - 363	
	50 g	96 h	287	T	F	15	7.9 - 8.2	358 - 363	Kumaraguru & Beamish (1981)
	200 g	96 h	314	T	F	15	7.9 - 8.2	358 - 363	
	6 cm, 3 g	24 h	135	T		10	7.5	110	Coats & O'Donnell-Jeffery (1979)
	6 cm, 3 g	24 h	61	EC		10	7.5	110	

Table 5 (contd).

Species	Size	Duration of test	Toxicity[a] (µg/litre)	Formulation[d]	System[e]	Temperature (°C)	pH	Hardness	Reference
Rainbow trout (contd).									
(Salmo gairdneri)	5 - 6 cm	48 h	6.0	EC		12			Mulla et al.
	5 - 6 cm	48 h	7.0	cis, EC		25.5			(1978a)
	2 - 4 g	24 h	18	T	S	12			Glickman
	2 - 4 g	24 h	25	cis	S	12			et al.
	2 - 4 g	24 h	14	trans	S	12			(1981)
Killifish	adult	48 h	41	T	S	25			Miyamoto (1976)
(Oryzias latipes)	adult	48 h	17	(+)-trans	S	25			Miyamoto (1976)
	adult	48 h	13	(+)-cis	S	25			Miyamoto (1976)
	adult	48 h	> 10 000	(-)-trans	S	25			Miyamoto (1976)
	adult	48 h	> 10 000	(-)-cis	S	25			Miyamoto (1976)
Channel catfish *(Ictalurus punctatus)*	1.4 - 1.7 cm, (0.02 g)	96 h	1.1	EC	S	24		100	Jolly et al. (1978)
Largemouth Bass *(Micropterus salmoides)*	4.5 - 5.5 cm, (1.14 g)	96 h	8.5	EC	S	24		100	Jolly et al. (1978)
Mosquitofish *(Gambusia affinis)*	1.5 - 2.5 cm, (0.25 g)	96 h	15	EC	S	24		100	Jolly et al. (1978)
	4 - 5 cm	48 h	97.0	EC		8.8 - 16			Mulla et al.
	4 - 5 cm	48 h	13.0	cis, EC		8.8 - 16			(1978a)
Brook trout *(Salvelinus foutinalis)*	1.2 g	96 h	3.2	T	S	12	7.5	40	Mayer & Ellersieck (1986)
Fathead minnow *(Pimephales promelas)*	0.6 g	96 h	5.7	T	S	22	7.3	38	Mayer & Ellersieck (1986)
Bluegill sunfish *(Lepomis macrochirus)*	0.7 g	96 h	5.0	T	S	22	7.3	38	Mayer & Ellersieck (1986)
Desert pupfish	4 - 5 cm	48 h	5.0	EC	S	11 - 16.5			Mulla et al.
(Cyprinodon macularis)	4 - 5 cm	48 h	5.0	cis, EC	S	11 - 16.5			(1978a)
Tilapia mossambica	5 - 6 cm	48 h	44.0	EC	S	15 - 21.4			Mulla et al.
	5 - 6 cm	48 h	5.6	cis, EC	S	15 - 21.4			(1978a)
Amphibian									
Bullfrog, tadpole *(Rana catesbeiana)*	0.6 - 0.8 cm	96 h	7033	EC	S	24		100	Jolly et al. (1978)

Table 5 (contd).

Species	Size	Duration of test	Toxicity[a] (µg/litre)	Formulation[d]	System[e]	Temperature (°C)	pH	Salinity (°/oo)	Reference
B. Estuarine and Marine Organisms									
Algae									
Skeletonema costatum		96 h	92[b]	T		20			Borthwich & Walsh *(1981)*
Molluscs									
Oyster *(Crassostrea virginica)*	2-h larva	48 h	> 1000[c]	T	S	25		20	Borthwich & Walsh *(1981)*
Arthropods									
Lobster *(Homarus americanus)*	450 g	96 h	0.73	T	R	10		30	McLeese et al. (1980)
Shrimp *(Crangon Septemspinosa)*	1.3 g	96 h	0.13	T	R	10			
Shrimp *(Mysidopsis bahia)*	1-day, juvenile	96 h	0.046	T	S	25		20	Borthwich & Walsh (1981)
Stone crab *(Menippe mercenaria)*	Zoea larva	96 h	0.018	T	S	25		20	
Pink shrimp *(Penaeus duorarum)*	adult	96 h	0.22	T	F	25		25	Mayer (1987)
Fish									
Harpacticoid *(Nitocra spinipes)*	3-6 weeks old	96 h	0.6	EC	S	20 - 22	7.8	7	Linden et al. (1979)
Bleak *(Alburnus alburnus)*	8 cm	96 h	4 - 8	EC	S	10	7.8	7	
Sheepshead minnow *(Cyprinodon variegatus)*	28-day fry	96 h	88	T	S	25		20	Borthwich & Walsh (1981)
	adult	96 h	7.8	T	F	30		22	Mayer (1987)
Atlantic silverside *(Menidia menidia)*	adult	96 h	2.2	T	F	26		25	Mayer (1987)
Striped mullet *(Mugil cephalus)*	juvenile	96 h	5.5	T	F	24		19	Mayer (1987)

a Values are LC_{50} unless stated otherwise.
b EC_{50} (growth inhibition).
c EC_{50} (abnormal development).
d T = Technical, EC = Emulsifiable concentrate.
e R = Renewal, S = Static, F = Flow-through.
f expressed as mg $CaCO_3$/litre.

When permethrin was sprayed at 8.8, 17.5, 35.0, or 70.0 g ai/ha by aeroplane over small trout streams, the impact on aquatic invertebrates and effects on the general fish population correlated with the dose. There was an increase in the number of organisms drifting downstream, the major ones being mayflies, followed by caddisflies, stoneflies, and chironomids. The total number of drifting organisms was greater than the pre-spray average by factors of 303, 699, 4960, and 6450 with spray concentrations of 8.8, 17.5, 35.0, and 70.0 g ai/ha, respectively. A return to pre-spray drift levels was evident within 36 h after application at 8.8 and 17.5 g ai/ha whereas drifting of organism persisted for up to 72 h at the higher application rates of 35 and 70 g ai/ha. Following the spraying of permethrin at these higher doses, there was no evidence of fish mortality, but there appeared a dramatic change in the diets of fish (such as the native brook trout and sculpins). These fish became virtually completely dependent on terrestrial invertebrates rather than on the aquatic insects for food. When the rate of application was low (8.8 g ai/ha) permethrin did not appear to affect these fish, either in mortality rate or in their diet composition (Kingsbury & Kreutzweiser, 1980b).

Serial applications of permethrin, once or twice at 17.5 g ai/ha, resulted in catastrophic drift of aquatic invertebrates and substantial depletion of benthos in streams within the application blocks and up to 2 km downstream. Despite massive disturbances of benthos, repopulation of bottom fauna was evident within 2.5 months and had virtually returned to normal within 3.5 months. Permethrin residues attained peak levels of 1.35 μg/litre in standing water and 1.94 μg/litre in flowing water in the sprayed regions. The residue persisted at low concentrations for up to 96 h after spraying (Kreutzweiser, 1982).

In a study by Kingsbury & Kreutzweiser (1987), aerial applications of permethrin to forests over several seasons at 8.8, 17.5, 35, and 70 g ai/ha did not cause mortality to native and caged fish (minnows, mudminnows, perch, and under-yearling and yearling Atlantic salmon). The composition of the salmonid diet was subsequently altered from aquatic insects (mayfly nymphs, stonefly nymphs, and various aquatic fly larvae) to terrestrial arthropods. The duration of changes ranged from a few months after applications of 8.8 and 17.5 g ai/ha to a year or longer after treatment with 35 and 70 g ai/ha. There were temporary reductions in fish growth rate and fish densities in the treated area, which returned to normal within four months after treatment. In the same study, the effect on stream invertebrates was also evaluated. Large drifts of invertebrates were observed immediately after applications and continued for 24 to 72 h. Although the peak of permethrin residues in stream water was higher after the second application (0.36-1.80 μg/litre) than the first (0.25-0.62 μg/litre), drift response to the second application ranged from 6 to 62% of the first drift, indicating that first application deleted susceptible invertebrates (e.g., *Ephemeroptera* nymphs, *Plecoptera*, *Trichoptera*, and the *Diptera* families) and that a much smaller residual population responded to the second treatment. Recovery of benthic fauna was apparent between 1 and 18 months after spraying. The double treatment reduced benthos density to a point at which recovery of numbers was slower than after the single application (Kreutzweiser & Kingsbury, 1987).

6.2 Toxicity to Terrestrial Organisms

6.2.1 Soil microorganisms

Mathur et al. (1980) applied permethrin (Ambush 5 G) to Canadian soils with a high content of organic material at a rate of 2.24 kg/ha. Lettuce or carrots were grown on the plots. Soil cores were taken at regular intervals and bacterial and fungal numbers were estimated, soil nutrients were measured, and acid phosphatase activity in the soil was monitored. Residues of permethrin persisted throughout the growing season up to crop harvest, when 65% of the original concentration in soil was found (113 days after application). This reflected the poor breakdown of permethrin in organic soils compared to mineral soils. Permethrin suppressed bacterial and actinomycete populations in samples taken 1, 9, and 27 days after application, but control levels were re-gained after 41 days (the next sampling time). The available nitrogen and phosphorus was lower in treated soil at some points during the study, but these changes were not consistent. Soil respiration and acid phosphatase activity were higher in permethrin-treated plots, though not consistently so. Permethrin had a greater effect when carrots were grown than when lettuce was grown. The yield of neither crop was affected. Most of the effects reported were transitory and none were of overall significance for either the soil or the crop.

6.2.2 Terrestrial invertebrates

Under laboratory conditions, permethrin is highly toxic to certain beneficial insects or natural enemies of pests, as shown in Table 6.

Cox & Wilson (1984) treated honey bee workers topically with a sub-lethal dose of permethrin (0.09 μg/bee in 1.0 μl of acetone applied to the thorax). This dose gave no higher mortality than treatment with acetone alone. The bees, which were individually tagged, were housed in an observation hive and trained before the experiment to feed at an artificial feeding station 5 m from the hive. The experiment was conducted at 35°C because at lower temperatures this dose resulted in mortality. Treated bees made less foraging trips than controls and gave food less frequently to other bees in the hive. Other behaviours were increased in treated bees, i.e., self-cleaning, trembling dance, ab-domen tucking, and rotating and cleaning of abdomen while rubbing the hind legs together. Gerig (1985) also reported minimal lethal effects on honey bees of permethrin used at recommended rates and that the insecticide had a strong repellent effect.

Pike et al. (1982) applied permethrin by helicopter at a rate of 0.22 kg ai/ha to fields of maize (*Zea mays*). The applications were made early in the morning before bees were actively foraging for pollen

Table 6. Acute toxicity of permethrin to non-target terrestrial organisms

Species	Size	Application	Duration	Toxicity[a]	Temperature (°C)	Reference
Bird						
Hen		oral		> 1.5 g/kg b.w.[b]		Millner & Butterworth (1977)
Chicken		oral		> 3 g/kg b.w.[b]		Worthing & Walker (1983)
Japanese quail		oral	5 days	> 13.5 g/kg b.w.[b]		Hill & Camardese (1986)
		diet	5 days	> 5 g/kg diet[c]		
		diet	5 days	> 5 g/kg diet[d]		
Mallard duck		diet	5 days	> 27.5 g/kg diet		Ross et al. (1976b)
Mallard duck		oral		> 13.5 g/kg b.w.[b]		Ross et al. (1976a)
Starling		diet	5 days	> 27.5 g/kg diet		Ross et al. (1976d)
Starling		oral		> 38 g/kg b.w.[b]		Ross et al. (1976c)
Ring-necked pheasant		diet	5 days	> 27.5 g/kg diet		Ross et al. (1976e)
Ring-necked pheasant		oral		> 13.5 g/kg b.w.[b]		Ross et al. (1977a)
Arthropods						
Honeybee *(Apis mellifera)*		contact		0.11 µg/bee[b]	26 - 27	Stevenson et al. (1978)
		oral		0.28 µg/bee[b]	26 - 27	Stevenson et al. (1978)
Insect parasite						
Ichneumoid *(Campoletis sonorensis)*	adult male	film	24 h	0.31 µg/vial		Plapp & Vinson (1977)

Table 6 (contd).

Species	Size	Application	Duration	Toxicity[a]	Temperature (°C)	Reference
Insect predator						
Carabid *(Pterostichus melanarius)*	adult 0.16 g	topical		> 2000 μg/insect[b]	21	Hagley et al. (1980)
Carabid *(Harpalus affinis)*	adult 0.05 g	topical		116 μg/insect[b]	21	Hagley et al. (1980)
Carabid *(Amara* sp.)	adult 0.03 g	topical		25 μg/insect[b]	21	Hagley et al. (1980)
Earwig *(Labidura raparia)*	mature	soil 0.1 kg ai/ha		6% mortality		Workman (1977)
	mature	soil 0.2 kg ai/ha		50% mortality		Workman (1977)
Green lacewing *(Chrysopa carnea)*	larvae 5-6 days old	film		9.87 μg/vial	25	Plapp & Bull (1978)
Predaceous mite species						
Mataseiulus occidentalis (3 strains)	adult female	slide-dip method		0.72, 1.32, 14.8 mg ai/litre	27.5	Roush & Hoy (1978)
	young gravid female	leaf-disc method		2.8 mg ai/litre	27	Hoy et al. (1979)
(Amblyseius fallacis)	adult female	slide-dip method		14 mg ai/litre	27	Rock (1979)

a LC_{50} values, unless stated otherwise.
b LD_{50} values; b.w. = body weight.
c Technical product.
d Emulsifiable concentrate.

and were repeated every 3 to 6 days (to a maximum of six applications per season). The trial was repeated for 3 years. There was no difference in the number of dead bees per hive between treated and control areas, but a marked reduction in the number of bees foraging in treated fields, indicating avoidance of permethrin. The authors concluded that treatment of corn fields with permethrin at the normal application rate is safe for bees as long as the application does not coincide with bee activity in the area.

The acute toxicity values of permethrin to tobacco budworm (*Heliothis virescens*), to the green lacewing (*Chrysopa carnea*), a predator of tobacco budworm, and to *Campoletis sonorensis*, an ichneumoid parasite of tobacco budworm, showed that permethrin was approximately 18 times less toxic to the predators than to the pest (Plapp & Bull, 1978; Plapp & Vinson, 1977).

Larvae of the green lacewing exhibited marked tolerance to permethrin, and to its cis or trans isomers, when dosed topically with 250 μg per insect (about 25 000 μg/g). This value is $\approx$10 000 times greater than the LD_{50} value for the tobacco budworm (Shour & Crowder, 1980).

Workman (1977) added permethrin to loamy sand soil into which the striped earwig (*Labidura riparia*), an effective insect predator of the cabbage looper, was introduced. The insecticide was of low toxicity to the earwig at dosage rates which gave good looper control.

The susceptibility of carabids to permethrin appears to be inversely related to beetle size, as shown in Table 6. When permethrin was applied at a concentration of 0.21-0.85 kg ai/ha to an apple orchard, it did not significantly affect the numbers of *Pterostichus melanarius* at any time during the season, but the numbers of *Harpalus affinis* and *Amara* sp. were significantly reduced 3-5 days after application. This result reflected the toxicity ratings by means of LD_{50} values obtained in laboratory studies. The total seasonal numbers of these carabids were not significantly affected by permethrin, owing to short residual effects (Hagley et al., 1980).

In laboratory tests, LC_{50} values of permethrin for two strains of spider mites (*Tetranychus urticae*) were $\approx$20-40 times greater than those for three strains of predator mites (*Mataseiulus occidentalis*) (Roush & Hoy, 1978), and $\approx$15 times greater than those for *Amblyseius fallacis* (Rock, 1979). These studies indicate that the use of permethrin at the recommended rates of 60-120 mg ai/litre would be detrimental to orchard integrated mite control programs.

In laboratory tests, the Pacific spider mite (*T. pacificus*) has been found to be 40 times more tolerant to permethrin than the predator mite (*M. occidentalis*), (Hoy et al., 1979). The spraying of vineyards with 15 or 30 mg ai/litre resulted in substantially higher populations of *T. pacificus* and *E. willamettei* for about one month due to reduction in predator species numbers. Similarly, spraying with 60 or 120 mg ai/litre produced a subsequent increase of *Eotetranychus willamettei* late in August and September for the above reason (Hoy et al., 1979).

When permethrin was applied to apple trees at a concentration of 40 mg/litre, no predator mites (*Typhlodromus pyri*) were found for 4-6 weeks, and only small numbers were found 10 weeks after the spray. On the other hand, permethrin had no appreciable toxicity to the spider mite (*Panonychus ulmi*). The virtual elimination of the predatory mite by permethrin spraying led to a marked population increase of *P. ulmi* later in the same season (Aliniazee & Cranham, 1980).

In apple and pear orchards, applications of permethrin at 30 mg ai/litre reduced the numbers of a predatory mite (*M. occidentalis*) to almost zero and dramatically increased the populations of spider mites (*T. urticae, Tetranychus mcdanieli*, or *P. ulmi*) (Hoyt et al., 1978).

From the above findings it appeared that permethrin, when applied according to recommendations, is relatively harmless to insect predators, with the exception of predaceous mite species. Everts et al. (1985) investigated the effects of permethrin on beneficial terrestrial arthropods in the soil and vegetation in areas surrounding applications of the insecticide to control tsetse flies in the Ivory Coast, West Africa. Permethrin was used as a 2.5% wettable powder at a rate of 121 g ai/ha during January (a minimum temperature of 20.0°C and a maximum of 36.0°C). The permethrin application significantly reduced populations of Coleoptera, Lepidoptera, Ephydridae, Chloropidae, Muscidae, Ichneumonidea, Chalcidoidea and Proctotrupoidea. The populations of almost all these groups were found to recover to normal levels within 2 months, i.e., before the likely time of respraying for the control of the tsetse flies. However, one Proctotrupoid genus, Cremastobaeus, was eliminated by permethrin treatment.

6.2.3 Birds

Neither an acute oral nor a dietary LD_{50} or LC_{50} has been established accurately because of the very low toxicity of permethrin to birds (Table 6). The acute LD_{50} is >3000 mg/kg body weight and the dietary toxicity >5000 mg/kg diet. (Worthing & Walker, 1983; Hill & Camardese, 1986).

The inclusion of permethrin at up to 40 mg/kg in the diet of laying hens for 28 days had no adverse effects on the health of parent birds or on egg production quality, hatchability, or the viability of the chicks produced (Ross et al. 1977b).

6.2.4 Mammals

Racey & Swift (1986) treated roosting boxes for pipistrelle bats with various wood preservatives and allowed the bats to roost in the boxes for up to 154 days. There were no toxic effects of mixtures of synthetic pyrethroids including permethrin. The authors concluded that the insecticide component of wood preservatives should be pyrethroids when bats are present in the area.

6.3 Uptake, Loss, Bioaccumulation and Biomagnification

Proposed metabolic pathways of permethrin in fish are summarized in Fig. 4.

When rainbow trout (*Salmo gairdneri*) were held in static water containing 5 μg/litre of ^{14}C-permethrin for 24 h, both cis and trans isomers were similarly taken up into the fish. The bioaccumulation ratios for total radiocarbon in the blood, muscle, liver, and fat of the fish were 30, 30, 300, and 400, respectively. When the fish were transferred to fresh running water, radioactivity was eliminated, with initial half-lives of 9-35 h, from all the tissues except fat, where little decay in ^{14}C-permethrin concentrations occurred. When rainbow trout were injected intraperitoneally with ^{14}C-permethrin at a rate of 0.5 mg/kg, 32-43% of the dose was recovered after 48 h in the bile, 3-7% in the urine, and 31-42% in the carcass. However, the urine and bile of the trout injected with the trans isomer contained higher levels of radioactivity. In the bile, the major metabolite was the glucuronide conjugate of 3-(4-hydroxyphenoxy)-benzyl-3-(2,2-dichlorovinyl)-2,2-dimethyl-cyclopropanecarboxylate (26) and there were few metabolites formed by hydrolysis (Fig. 4). The urine contained principally the sulfate conjugates of polar products. The ability of rainbow trout to hydrolyze permethrin *in vivo* appeared minimal (Glickman et al., 1981).

The rates of *trans*-permethrin hydrolysis in trout liver, kidney, and plasma incubated at 12°C were approximately 166, 38, and 59 times, respectively, lower than those in the corresponding mouse tissues incubated at 37°C. Although an increase in the incubation temperature from 12°C to 37°C caused an increase in the rate of *trans*-permethrin hydrolysis by trout liver microsomes, *trans*-permethrin was hydrolyzed about 45 times slower than by mouse liver microsomes at 37°C. The hydrolysis of permethrin in trout plasma, however, was higher than that in trout liver microsomes (Glickman & Lech, 1981).

When the microsomal preparations of both carp and rainbow trout were fortified with NADPH, the carp microsomes oxidized permethrin isomers more actively than the trout microsomes. Also, larger amounts of hydroxy ester metabolites were recovered with the cis isomer than with the trans isomer. The preferred site of oxidation of both isomers by the carp and trout microsomes was the 4′-position (26) of the phenoxybenzyl moiety. The geminal dimethyl group was attacked in preference to the methyl group situated trans to the carboxy group. *trans*-Permethrin primarily underwent hydrolysis by both carp and trout liver microsomes in the presence or absence of NADPH to yield PBalc (6) and Cl_2CA (17) (Glickman et al., 1979). In this respect, the results of *in vitro* studies were different from those obtained *in vivo*.

Juvenile Atlantic salmon (lipid content 4.2%), exposed for 96 h to static water containing 22 μg/litre permethrin, took up the insecticide with a bioaccumulation ratio of 55. Dead juvenile salmon exposed for 12.5 h to 0.098-0.994 mg/litre contained 2.21-3.69 μg/g (Zitko et al., 1977).

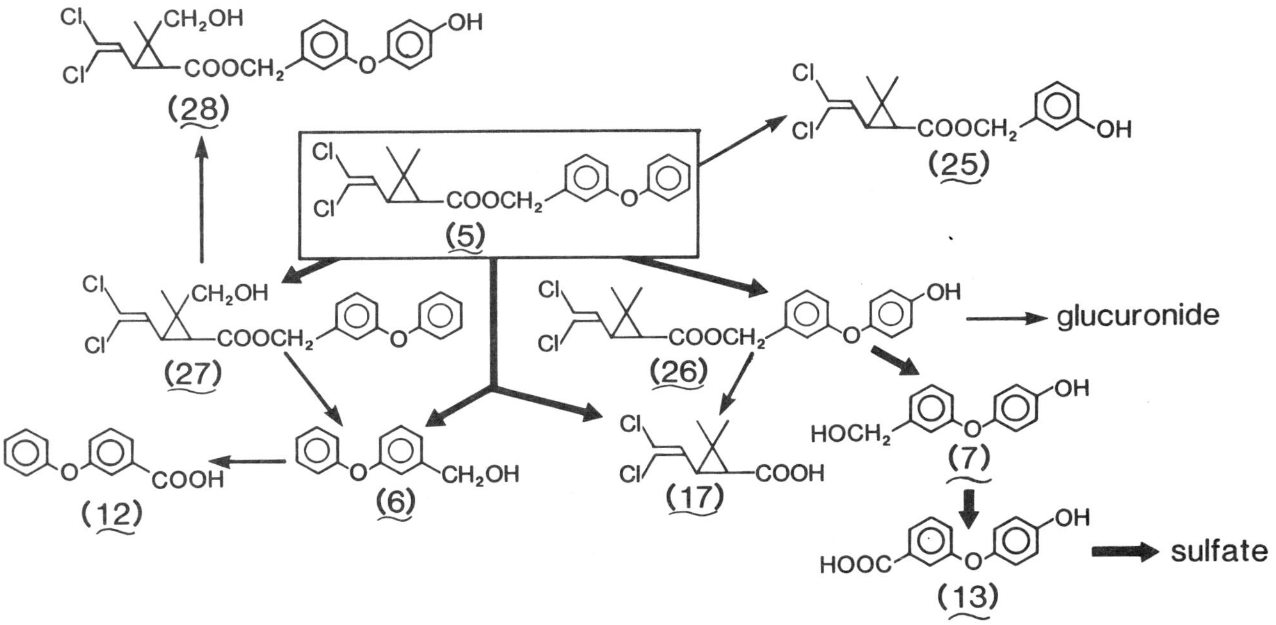

Fig. 4. Proposed metabolic pathways for permethrin in fish.

Residues of approximately 0.5-1.2 mg/kg were detected in dead juvenile Atlantic salmon exposed for 10-89 h to static water containing permethrin at 6.9-85 μg/litre, the bioaccumulation ratio ranging from 14 to 73. The insecticide was not detected (detection limit 5 ng/g) in dead lobster hepatopancreas or in dead shrimp (McLeese et al., 1980).

When stoneflies (*Pteronarcys dorsata*) were exposed for 28 days to running water containing permethrin at 0.029-0.21 mg/litre, the bioaccumulation ratios of the survivors ranged from 43 to 570 (average, 183; standard deviation, 171) (Anderson, 1982).

When carp were exposed to a ^{14}C-permethrin isomer (phenoxyphenyl-labelled [1R,trans], [1R,cis], [1S,trans], or [1S,cis] isomers) in a flow-through system at 25°C, the concentrations of ^{14}C and permethrin isomers in the fish body reached an equilibrium on days 7-9 of exposure. The bioaccumulation ratios of the permethrin isomers at equilibrium were 330-750. When the fish were transferred to fresh water, the permethrin isomers, as well as their metabolites, were rapidly excreted. The biological half-lives for the permethrin isomers were 2.0-2.8 days. The major metabolic reactions involved were oxidation at the 4′-position of the alcohol moiety or the methyl group of the acid moiety, cleavage of the ester linkage, and conjugation of the resultant alcohols and phenols with glucuronic acid or sulfuric acid (Ohshima et al., 1988).

Bioconcentration factors for sheepshead minnows (*Cyprinodon variegatus* exposed to permethrin at concentrations between 1.25 and 10 μg/litre for 28 days from hatching varied between 290 and 620. Maximum bioconcentration occurred after exposure at 2.5 μg/litre, and a maximum residue of 5.7 mg/kg occurred after exposure at 10 μg/litre (the concentrations were for whole fish) (Hansen et al., 1983).

Permethrin and its metabolites are not accumulated in birds. During repeated dosing to quails and to mallard ducks, very similar patterns and levels of both the appearance and depletion of radioactive residue in tissues were found. The level in fat, which was small, reached a plateau during a 28-day period. In all tissues, residues declined extensively during a 14-day period after the final dose (Leahey et al., 1977).

7. EFFECTS ON EXPERIMENTAL ANIMALS AND *IN VITRO* TEST SYSTEMS

Toxicological profiles of permethrins with different isomeric compositions (cis:trans ratios of 40:60 or 25:75) were compared in a range of toxicological studies. The toxicological profile of permethrin (25:75) resembles that of permethrin (40:60) except that it is less acutely toxic than permethrin (40:60).

7.1 Acute Toxicity

Table 7 shows the results of acute toxicity tests of permethrin with various animal species. Aqueous suspensions usually produced the least toxic results, LD_{50} values ranging from 3000 to >4000 mg/kg body weight. However, corn oil is the more standard vehicle for pyrethroids and yielded LD_{50} values of about 500 mg/kg (in all studies except one) for oral administration in rats and mice.

Following oral administration of permethrin to rats, signs of poisoning became apparent within 2 h after dosing and persisted for up to 3 days. At lethal levels, these signs included whole body tremors of varying degree from slight to convulsive, which in some cases were accompanied by salivation. Associated signs were hyperactivity and hyperexcitability to external stimuli, urination and defecation, ataxia, and lacrimation (Parkinson, 1978; Litchfield, 1983).

Table 8 gives the acute oral toxicity of three lots of permethrin to rats. The observed ten-fold decrease in LD_{50} when corn oil or olive oil were used could be due to enhanced absorption of the insecticide (Metker et al, 1977).

The acute oral toxicity of permethrin (25:75) to groups of six female C.S.E. Wistar rats was determined in five different vehicles (Table 9). Most symptoms of acute poisoning developed within 12 h of dosing and consisted of muscular tremors, hypersensitivity to stimuli, and staining of abdominal fur. The majority of deaths occurred between 1 and 3 days (Wallwork & Malone, 1974).

Groups of female Sprague-Dawley rats, either fed *ad libitum* or starved for 24 h beforehand, were given a single oral dose of permethrin (25:75) (94.1% purity) in corn oil solution (40% w/v) at 750, 1500, 3000, or 6000 mg/kg. Permethrin was more toxic in starved animals (LD_{50} = 3000 mg/kg) than in animals that had been fed (LD_{50} = 4251 mg/kg) (Piercy et al., 1976).

The acute toxicity of permethrin with various *cis*- and *trans*-permethrin ratios is indicated in Table 10. These data clearly demonstrate that *cis*-permethrin is more toxic than *trans*-permethrin to rats and mice.

Table 7. Acute toxicity of permethrin administered to various animal species

Species	Sex	Route[a]	Vehicle[b]	LD_{50} (mg/kg body weight)	Reference
Rat	M	oral	water[c]	2949	Parkinson 1978
	F	oral	water	> 4000	Parkinson et al. 1976
	M	oral	DMSO	1500	Clark 1978
	F	oral	DMSO	1000	Clark 1978
	M	oral	corn oil	500	Jaggers & Parkinson 1979
	M	oral	corn oil	430	Kohda et al. 1979a
	F	oral	corn oil	470	Kohda et al. 1979a
	M&F	oral	corn oil	1200	Braun & Killeen 1975
	M&F	oral	water	1725	Sasinovich & Panshina 1987
	M	dermal	water	> 5176	Parkinson 1978
	F	dermal	none[d]	> 4000	Parkinson et al. 1976
	M	dermal	none[d]	> 2500	Kohda et al. 1979a
	F	dermal	none[d]	> 2500	Kohda et al. 1979a
	M&F	dermal	xylene	> 750	Clark 1978
	M&F	dermal	none	2000	Sasinovich & Panshina 1987
	M	sc	corn oil	7800	Kohda et al. 1979a
	F	sc	corn oil	6600	Kohda et al. 1979a
	M	ip	water	> 3200	Parkinson et al. 1976
	F	ip	water	> 3200	Parkinson et al. 1976
		ip		463 - 1725	Sasinovich & Panshina 1987
Mouse	F	oral	water	> 4000	Parkinson et al. 1976
	M&F	oral	DMSO	250 - 500	Clark 1978
	M	oral	corn oil	650	Kohda et al. 1979a
	F	oral	corn oil	540	Kohda et al. 1979a
	M	dermal	none[d]	> 2500	Kohda et al. 1979a
	F	dermal	none[d]	> 2500	Kohda et al. 1979a
	M	sc	corn oil	> 10 000	Kohda et al. 1979a
	F	sc	corn oil	10 000	Kohda et al. 1979a
Rabbit	F	oral	water[c]	> 4000	Parkinson et al. 1976
	F	dermal	none[d]	> 2000	Parkinson et al. 1976
Guinea-pig	M	oral	water	> 4000	Parkinson et al. 1976
Hen		oral		> 1500	Milner & Butterworth 1977

[a] sc = subcutaneous; ip = intraperitoneal.

[b] DMSO = dimethyl sulfoxide.

[c] as an aqueous suspension.

[d] technical material applied without vehicle.

Table 8. Acute oral toxicity of three lots of permethrin to rats

Lot No.[c]	Strain	Sex	Solvent	LD_{50} (mg/kg)
827-RSP-1422	Sprague-Dawley	Male Female	None None	5010 3801
827-RTP-1450	Sprague-Dawley-1[a]	Male	Corn oil	563
	Sprague-Dawley-2[b]	Male	Corn oil	383
827-RTP-1450	Long-Evans	Male Female	None None	4892 2712
8719-RTP-1450	Sprague-Dawley	Male Female	Olive oil Corn oil	584 413

[a] Average body weight was 220 g.
[b] Average body weight was 321 g.
[c] Isomeric composition and the purity of the compound in each lot were as follows:

Lot No.	Isomeric Ratio cis	Isomeric Ratio trans	Stated Purity
827-RSP-1422	44%	56%	93.6%
827-RTP-1450	45%	55%	95.0%
8719-RTP-1450	46.5%	53.5%	92.4%

Table 9. Acute toxicity of permethrin (25:75) to rats

Vehicle	LD_{50} (mg/kg)
Neat undiluted permethrin (control)	> 20 000
40% w/v in corn oil	4672
40% w/v in petroleum distillate	> 8000
40% w/v in dimethylsulfoxide	> 8000
20% w/v in glycerol	> 5048

Table 10. Acute toxicity of permethrins with various cis:trans isomeric ratios

Permethrin (cis:trans)	Animal	Sex	Route[a]	LD_{50} (mg/kg body weight)	Reference
80:20	Rat	F	oral	396	Jaggers & Parkinson (1979)
57:43		F	oral	333	
50:50		F	oral	748	
40:60		F	oral	630	
20:80		F	oral	2800	
99:1	Mouse		ip	108	Glickman et al. (1982)
40:60			ip	514	
1:99			ip	> 800	
99:1	Mouse		iv	17	Glickman et al. (1982)
40:60			iv	31	
1:99			iv	> 135	

[a] ip = intraperitoneal; iv = intravenous.

Table 11 shows the results of acute oral toxicity tests of the metabolites of permethrin on rats (FAO/WHO, 1980b).

Table 11. Acute oral toxicity to rats of several metabolites of permethrin

Chemical	No.[a]	LD_{50} (mg/kg body weight)
3-phenoxybenzyl alcohol	6	1330
3-(2,2-dichlorovinyl)-2,2-dimethylcyclo-propanecarboxylic acid	17	980
3-phenoxybenzaldehyde	11	600

[a] Chemical identification no. used in Fig. 3.

Table 12 shows the results of the acute intraperitoneal toxicity to mice of permethrin metabolites (Kohda et al., 1979b).

Table 12. Acute intraperitoneal toxicity to mice of several permethrin metabolites

Chemical[a]	No.[b]	LD_{50} (mg/kg body weight)	
		Male	Female
3-phenoxybenzyl alcohol	6	71	424
3-(4′-hydroxyphenoxy)benzyl alcohol	7	750 - 1000	750 - 1000
3-(2′-hydroxyphenoxy)benzyl alcohol	8	876	778
3-phenoxybenzoic acid	12	154	169
3-(4′-hydroxyphenoxy)benzoic acid	13	783	745
3-(2′-hydroxyphenoxy)benzoic acid	14	859	912
3-phenoxybenzaldehyde	11	415	416

[a] All compounds were dissolved in corn oil, except 3-phenoxybenzoic acid, which was dissolved in DMSO.
[b] Chemical identification no. used in Fig. 3.

7.2 Subacute and Subchronic Toxicity

7.2.1 Oral exposure

7.2.1.1 Mouse

When male and female Alderly Park mice (20 of each sex per group) were fed permethrin in the diet at levels of 0, 200, 400, 2000, or 4000 mg/kg diet for 28 days, mortality, growth, and food utilization were normal for all animals. One additional group (permethrin level of 80 mg/kg for 2 weeks and 10 000 mg/kg for the final 2 weeks) showed weight loss and poor food utilization when feeding with 10 000 mg/kg began. Animals fed permethrin at 2000 mg/kg or more showed increased liver weight and liver-to-body weight ratio. Higher weight and organ-to-body weight ratios were also observed in the kidney, heart, and spleen of males receiving a dose of 10 000 mg/kg. Gross tissue changes were observed in females at 2000 and 10 000 mg/kg. On histopathological examination, regenerating tubules in the renal cortex and hypertrophy of centrilobular hepatocytes with cytoplasmic eosinophilia, which were not dose related, were observed in all the treated animals (Clapp et al., 1977b).

In a study by Wallwork et al. (1974a), groups of six mature female mice received daily oral doses of permethrin (25:75) in corn oil at 0, 200, 400, 800, or 1600 mg/kg body weight for 10 consecutive days. Signs of acute toxicity, such as spasm and convulsion, were seen only in the highest dose group, half of which died after the initial dose. No significant changes in haematology, clinical chemistry, or body weights on the 11th day of dosing were recorded. The mice treated at 800 and 1600 mg/kg body weight exhibited increased liver weights.

7.2.1.2 Rat

Sprague-Dawley rats (six of each sex per group) were fed permethrin in the diet for 14 days at dose levels of 54, 108, 216, 432, 864, or 1728 mg/kg body weight per day. All rats surviving to term were sacrificed and various organs and tissues were examined histopathologically. At the two highest dose levels, all animals died except one female fed 864 mg/kg. Muscle tremors were noted in all animals at 432 mg/kg, but doses of 216 mg/kg or less caused no toxic signs in either males or females. There was a statistically significant increase in average liver-to-body weight ratios at 432 mg/kg, but compound-related histological changes were not observed in any of the tissues or organs. The maximum NOEL in this study was 216 mg/kg (Metker et al., 1977).

In studies by Metker et al. (1977), Long-Evans rats (six of each sex per group) were fed permethrin in the diet for 14 days at dose levels of 0, 27, 54, 108, 216, or 432 mg/kg body weight per day. All rats surviving to term were sacrificed and various organs and tissues were examined histopathologically. At a dose of 432 mg/kg, three out of six females died within the first five days. Muscle tremors were noted in all surviving animals at 216 and 432 mg/kg. There was a statistically significant increase among female animals in the average liver-to-body weight ratio. Compound-related histological changes were not observed in any of the tissues or organs examined. The maximum dietary NOEL was 108 mg/kg body weight per day.

When young male and female Wistar rats (8 of each sex per group) were fed permethrin in the diet at dose levels of 0, 200, 500, 1000, 2500, 5000, or 10 000 mg/kg diet for 4 weeks, all rats that received the highest dose died within 3 days. Mortality was evident at 5000 mg/kg, and hyperexcitability was observed in animals that received 2500 mg/kg. Other non-specific signs of poisoning were observed at 1000 mg/kg on the first day of the study only. Food consumption and growth were reduced in the animals dosed at 5000 mg/kg. There was no effect on haematological parameters, clinical chemistry, or urinalysis except for a reduction in urinary protein excretion in males at 5000 mg/kg. Liver weight and liver-to-body weight ratios were increased in males at 2500 mg/kg or more and in females at 1000 mg/kg or more. This study had been designed as a preliminary range-finding test for long-term dietary administration (Clapp et al., 1977a).

In a study of the reversibility of hepatic changes in rats following short-term dietary administration of permethrin, female Wistar rats (48 rats per group) were fed permethrin at levels of 0 or 2500 mg/kg diet for 28 days. At the end of the feeding trial, rats were either sacrificed or maintained on control diets and sacrificed at 1, 4, or 8 weeks after the termination of dosing. There was no mortality, but food consumption, food utilization, and body weight were reduced in the permethrin-treated rats during the administration period. However, the animals gained weight rapidly after the dosing period and there was no difference in body weight between control and test animals at the end of the study period. After the 4 weeks of permethrin dosing, significantly higher absolute and relative liver weights were observed. During the 8-week recovery period, the relative liver weight of permethrin-treated animals was significantly higher than the control values, but the absolute weights of the liver of control and test animals were similar. There were no effects of permethrin on plasma alanine transaminase over the course of the study. Oxidative enzyme activity in liver microsomes was significantly higher in test animals than in controls at the end of dosing and 1 week later. The activity of liver microsomal enzymes in the permethrin-treated animals was normal 4 weeks after dosing but was elevated 8 weeks after dosing. The amount of smooth endoplasmic reticulum in rat liver cells was significantly increased as a result of permethrin dosing, but within 4 weeks after dosing, there were no significant histological differences in the liver between treated and control animals (Bradbrook et al., 1977).

When male and female Charles River (CD) rats (six of each sex per group) were fed permethrin at levels of 0, 30, 100, 300, 1000, or 3000 mg/kg diet for five weeks, persistent tremors were evident in animals fed at 3000 mg/kg although no mortality was observed. Growth was inhibited in both males and females at this dose level. Relative liver weight was increased in both the males (1000 mg/kg or more) and females (3000 mg/kg). Slight effects on certain clinical chemistry parameters, such as increased prothrombin times in males, were noted at the 3000 mg/kg level. Examination of tissues and organs of the animals receiving the two highest doses did not show any unusual effects as a result of permethrin in the diet (Butterworth & Hend, 1976).

Male and female Long-Evans rats (10 of each sex per group) fed permethrin in the diet at dose levels of 0, 20, 100, or 500 mg/kg diet for 90 days showed no mortality, and the growth and food consumption of all animals were normal. The results of haematology, clinical chemistry, urinalysis, and ophthalmological examinations were also normal. Tremors were noted in some animals at the highest dose level, mainly during the first week of treatment. There were significant increases in absolute and relative liver weights at the two highest dose levels. These increases were consistent with data from microscopic examination of the liver showing compound-related centrilobular hepatocyte hypertrophy in both males and females. There were no significant effects at the 20-mg/kg level, although slight hepatic effects were reported in a few of the male rats (Killeen & Rapp., 1976b).

In studies by Metker et al. (1977), Sprague-Dawley rats (10 of each sex per group) were fed permethrin in the diet for 90 days at dose levels of 0, 9, 27, 85, 270, or 850 mg/kg body weight per day. All rats surviving to term were killed and various tissues and organs from each animal were examined histopathologically. At 850 mg/kg, all male and female rats died. An increase in the average liver-to-body weight ratio was noted in both male and female rats fed 270 mg/kg. Compound-related histological changes were not observed in any of the tissues and organs examined. The minimum effect level was 270 mg/kg per day. At 85 mg/kg no effects were observed.

When male and female Sprague-Dawley rats (16 of each sex per group) were fed permethrin in the diet at dose levels of 0, 375, 750, 1500, or 3000 mg/kg diet for 6 months, there was no mortality and all animals exhibited normal growth and normal food and water consumption. Urinalysis, haematological values, and clinical biochemistry parameters showed no changes related to permethrin dosing. Signs of hyperexcitability and tremors were observed during the study in animals dosed at 3000 mg/kg and the liver weight and liver-to-body weight ratio of these animals were slightly increased. There were no significant histopathological findings attributable to the presence of the permethrin in the diet. The NOEL was 1500 mg/kg (Kadota et al., 1975).

In a study designed to evaluate liver hypertrophy, male and female Wistar rats were fed permethrin at levels of 0, 20, 100, or 1000 mg/kg diet for 26 weeks. There was no mortality, and the growth and food consumption of the animals were normal. Although the mean liver weight was increased at all dose levels, a significant increase was noted only at the highest dose level. The increase in liver weight at this dose level was accompanied by an increase in the smooth endoplasmic reticulum and in biochemical parameters associated with microsomal oxidative mechanisms. At a dose level of 100 mg/kg, there were slight, non-significant increases in biochemical activities. No effects on any of the parameters measured were observed in animals dosed at 20 mg/kg (Hart et al., 1977c).

In a study by Wallwork et al. (1974b), groups of five to six female Charles River CDI rats received permethrin (25:75) in corn oil at 0, 200, 400, or 800 mg/kg body weight by daily gavage for 10 days. The animals were sacrificed on the eleventh day so that haematological and clinical chemical parameters and organ weights could be investigated. Permethrin (25:75) gave a toxicity profile similar to that of permethrin (40:60).

7.2.1.3 Dog

Beagle dogs (four of each sex per group) fed permethrin in gelatin capsules daily for 3 months at dose levels of 0, 5, 50, or 500 mg/kg body weight showed no mortality, but clinical signs of poisoning were noted at various times in both males and females at the highest dose level. Growth and food consumption, as well as clinical chemical, haematological, and urinalysis parameters, were normal. The liver weights and liver-to-body weight ratios of animals that received permethrin at 50 mg/kg or more were significantly increased. Histopathological examination did not reveal any changes attributable to permethrin (Killeen & Rapp, 1976a).

Beagle dogs (four of each sex per group) administered permethrin in gelatin capsules daily for 13 weeks at dose levels of 0, 10, 100, and 2000 mg/kg body weight likewise showed no mortality, but clinical signs of poisoning were evident at 2000 mg/kg. Haematological, clinical chemical, and urinalysis values were normal in all animals. There was a slight increase in the liver weight of animals dosed at 2000 mg/kg/day, but no accompanying histopathological changes in the liver (Edwards et al., 1976).

When two beagle dogs were given daily oral doses of permethrin (25:75) at 500 mg/kg body weight for 14 days, there were no clinical signs of toxicity or significant effects of the treatment on body weight or on clinical chemistry or haematological parameters (Chesher et al., 1975a).

Groups of four male and four female beagle dogs, given encapsulated permethrin [(25:75) 4.5% w/v] at 0, 10, 50, or 250 mg/kg body weight for 6 months, revealed no signs of toxicity and no effect on body weight. Ophthalmoscopy and electrocardiography showed no abnormalities. At necropsy, there were no gross pathological or significant histopathological findings. Haematological and clinical chemistry parameters, including plasma antipyrine elimination rate, were unaffected by treatment. The results of this study indicate that daily oral doses up to 250 mg/kg body weight do not adversely affect beagle dogs (Reynolds et al., 1978).

7.2.1.4 Rabbits

In a study by Chesher & Malone (1974a), groups of five female Dutch rabbits received permethrin (25:75) in 10 daily doses by gavage in corn oil at 0, 200, 400, or 800 mg/kg body weight. The animals were killed on the eleventh day so that clinical chemical, haematological parameters, and organ weights could be investigated. One rabbit, dosed at 400 mg/kg, exhibited mild hyperactivity and muscular fasciculation, but only at days 6 and 7. Although all animals, including the controls, exhibited some degree of weight loss, it was most marked in the high-dose group. There were no significant haematological or clinical chemistry findings, but there was some decrease in liver and kidney weight and also some enlargement of adrenal gland weights in all treated groups.

7.2.1.5 Cow

Lactating cows (three per group) fed permethrin in the diet at dose levels of 0, 0.2, 1.0, 10, or 50 mg/kg diet for 28 days showed no mortality. Growth and milk production were normal, and no histopathological changes in the tissues were observed (Edwards & Iswaran, 1977).

7.2.2 Dermal Exposure

Technical grade permethrin was applied daily to the clipped skin of New Zealand White rabbits (eight males per group) at dose levels of 0, 0.10, 0.32, or 1.0 g/kg body weight, each day for 21 consecutive days. The application site was abraded on the first test day in half of the animals in each group. Blood samples were drawn weekly from the animals for clinical chemistry studies. All animals were killed on the tenth day after exposure ceased. Various tissues and organs were taken from each animal and examined for microscopic lesions. A moderate primary irritation of the skin was produced by permethrin. No significant changes in body weight, organ weight, or clinical chemistry values were evident, neither were there any compound-related lesions in the skin or other tissues (Metker et al., 1977).

In further studies by Metker et al. (1977), permethrin (dissolved in acetone) or acetone (as a control) was placed on the skin twice a week for 3 weeks to 6 groups of 10 shaved male New Zealand White rabbits. Cotton cloth treated with permethrin (1.25 or 0.125 mg/cm^2) was applied to the skin over 1 ml of artificial sweat (salt solution imitating sweat). In the case of other rabbits, similarly treated, the sweat was omitted. In the control groups, acetone-treated cotton cloth with or without 1 ml of sweat was used. Blood samples were collected once a week for clinical chemistry determinations. All animals surviving to term were killed and various tissues and organs from each animal were examined for microscopic lesions. No significant changes were noted in rabbit body weight or organ-to-body weight at the end of the 21-day test, and no skin irritation was observed. There were no significant changes in clinical chemistry values in the treated groups and no compound-related lesions in the skin or other tissues and organs examined (Metker et al., 1977).

7.2.3 Inhalation exposure

The inhalation toxicity of technical grade permethrin was determined in three species of laboratory animals. Male Hartley guinea-pigs, male and female Sprague-Dawley rats, and male and female beagle dogs were exposed to an aerosol of permethrin at concentrations of 125, 250, or 500 mg/m^3, 6 h per day, 5 days per week for 13 weeks. The mass median diameter of the aerosol droplets was 5.1 μm, and 85% of the total droplets had a diameter of 1.0 μm or less. At 500 mg/m^3, tremors and convulsions occurred in the rats during the first week of exposure but disappeared in the second week. There was no difference in oxygen consumption between control and treated rats. Urine metabolite studies indicated that permethrin was rapidly metabolized and excreted. Post-exposure experiments in male rats showed that the hexobarbital-induced sleeping time was significantly shortened after exposures at 500 mg/m^3 but not at lower doses. No clinical signs of poisoning were observed in the guinea-pigs and dogs when exposed to aerosols of permethrin under similar conditions. Pulmonary function, clinical chemistry parameters, and blood cell counts were unaffected in the beagle dogs following exposure. No compound-related gross or microscopic pathological changes or other permanent changes were observed in the dogs, rats, or guinea-pigs as a result of permethrin inhalation (Metker, 1978).

7.3 Primary Irritation

7.3.1 Skin irritation

When undiluted technical permethrin (91.3% purity, 0.5 ml) was applied to the clipped dorsal surface of Japanese White rabbits, there was no irritation (Okuno et al., 1976).

Single applications of 0.05 ml of 25% (w/v) permethrin (in 95% ethanol) or 10% (w/v) oil of bergamot solution (in 95% ethanol) (positive control) were applied to the intact skin of six rabbits. Five minutes later, some of the rabbits were exposed to UV light (365 nm) at a distance of 10-15 cm for 30 min (the intensity of UV light was not mentioned). Skin treated with the positive control solution and irradiated exhibited a greater irritation reaction than did non-irradiated skin. Permethrin did not cause any irritation reaction under the test conditions with or without irradiation (Metker et al., 1977).

When a permethrin formulation was applied to the clipped dorsal surface (0.13 mg/cm^2) of six New Zealand White rabbits (three of each sex) once a day for 16 days, a slight erythema appeared, which correlated with increased cutaneous blood flow measured by laser Doppler velocimetry. No significant histopathological changes were detected (Flannigan et al., 1985a).

7.3.2 Eye irritation

In a study by Okuno et al. (1976), 0.1 ml of undiluted technical permethrin (91.3% purity) was applied to the eyes of Japanese White rabbits. The eyes were washed with distilled water 5 min or 24 h after the application of permethrin. No eye irritation was observed.

Undiluted permethrin applied to the eyes of female rabbits caused minimal pain, redness, chemosis of the conjunctiva, and a slight discharge (Parkinson et al., 1976).

Permethrin (25:75) (40% in corn oil) did not produce any ocular effects when 0.1 ml was instilled into the ocular sac of New Zealand rabbits (Chesher & Malone, 1974c).

7.4 Sensitization

In a study by Parkinson et al. (1976), guinea-pigs were dermally administered permethrin as a 10% solution in dimethylformamide for 3 consecutive days. This was followed 4 days later by challenge doses of 0.1%, 1%, and 10% solutions of permethrin in dimethylformamide. Only very slight erythema was observed. Permethrin was therefore considered to be either non-sensitizing or only mildly so.

Guinea-pigs (10 per group) were initially injected intradermally with 0.1 ml permethrin solution and 14 days later were challenged with an intradermal injection (0.1 ml) of either a 0.1% solution of permethrin or dinitrochlorobenzene (DNCB). Five other animals per group received intradermally a challenge dose of 0.1% permethrin or DNCB without a prior sensitizing dose. The positive control substance (DNCB) elicited sensitization reactions in all guinea-pigs when examined 24 and 48 h after the challenge dose, whereas permethrin did not cause any sensitization reactions (Metker et al., 1977; Metker, 1978).

Permethrin (25:75) in corn oil (1% w/v) or Freund's complete adjuvant (1% w/v) did not produce dermal irritation or sensitization in groups of 10 male guinea-pigs when applied as a 25% dispersion in petrolatum. The positive control, DNCB, (5% w/v) in petrolatum produced marked sensitization (Chesher & Malone, 1974b).

7.5 Long-term Toxicity

7.5.1 Mouse

SPF Alderly Park strain mice (70 males and 70 females per group) were fed permethrin (cis 35-45%; trans 65-55%) at dose levels of 0, 250, 1000, or 2500 mg/kg diet for 2 years. Ten males and ten females were designated for interim kills at 26 and 52 weeks. The mortality rate was unaffected by the administration of permethrin. Growth was slightly decreased at the two highest dose levels at various periods during the study. At the interim sacrifice of 52 weeks and at the end of study, a significant dose-dependent increase in liver-to-body weight ratio was observed at the two highest dose levels in females (with 2500 mg/kg only at the end of the study) and at the highest dose level in males. Hepatic aminopyrine *N*-demethylase activity was also substantially increased, although not consistently, in both male and female mice given the highest dose. Gross and microscopic examination of tissues and organs (and specific examination for hepatic neoplasia) did not reveal any significant carcinogenic effects as a result of permethrin administration. Many of the non-tumour abnormalities observed were considered to be those associated with aging of the mice, characterized by increased eosinophilia of the centrilobular hepatocytes. Also, a decrease in vacuolation of the proximal tubular epithelium of the kidney was noted at all dietary levels in males. A high incidence of lung adenomas was observed with all animals in the study, but statistical analysis suggested that this was not related to permethrin feeding. Electron-microscopic examination of subcellular liver components showed a proliferation of the smooth endoplasmic reticulum at dose levels of 1000 and 2500 mg/kg. No notable effects on the sciatic nerve were found as the result of permethrin administration (Ishmael & Litchfield, 1988).

In studies by Hogan & Rinehart (1977) and Rapp (1978), CD-1 strain mice (75 of each sex per group) were fed permethrin in the diet for 104 weeks. Alterations were made in the dietary dose levels during the course of the study. From weeks 1 to 19, the animals were given dose levels of 0, 20, 100, and 500 mg/kg diet. At week 19, the dose level of 500 mg/kg was increased to 5000 mg/kg and maintained for 2 weeks before returning to 500 mg/kg. At week 21, the 100 mg/kg dose was increased to 4000 mg/kg and maintained for the remainder of the dosing period. Growth was inhibited in males at 4000 mg/kg. With the exception of a reduced blood glucose level in the animals receiving 4000 mg/kg, dietary administration of permethrin had no other effects on haematology or clinical chemistry parameters in the mouse. The liver weight was higher than it was in control animals in both male and female animals at a dose level of 500 mg/kg or more. In addition, the heart weight was higher at 4000 mg/kg. Neoplastic changes, not associated with dietary levels of permethrin, were observed in some animals in all groups. While there was no direct effect with respect to hepatic neoplasms, it was noted that hepatocellular hypertrophy, pleomorphism, and degeneration occurred in treated mice with increased frequency and appeared to show a dose-response relationship. No oncogenic effects were observed in the test animals.

7.5.2 Rat

Wistar rats (60 of each sex per group) were fed permethrin in the diet at dose levels of 0, 500, 1000, or 2500 mg/kg diet for 2 years, and twelve rats of each sex per group were sacrificed at 1 year. Signs of poisoning such as tremors and hyperexcitability were noted during the first 2 weeks of dosing in the animals that received the highest dose. There was no mortality attributable to permethrin, and growth and food consumption were unaffected. There were no effects on haematological, ophthalmological, urological, or other clinical chemistry parameters. Liver aminopyrine *N*-demethylase activity was increased in all permethrin-treated animals. Bone marrow smears of the animals showed no unusual findings. Gross and microscopic examination of tissues and organs was performed after 1 and 2 years, and all animals that died with neoplastic changes were examined. Liver weights were higher after 1 year of dosing in male and female rats that received permethrin at 2500 mg/kg than in the control animals. After 2 years, the liver weight and liver-to-body weight ratios were higher in all permethrin-treated males than in the corresponding controls. In the females, higher values of absolute and relative liver weights, compared to the controls, were recorded only in the group of animals dosed at 1000 mg/kg. Kidney weight was also increased, predominantly in males, at all dose levels. Hepatocyte vacuolation was seen at 1 year in males fed at the highest dose level only and in females at all dose levels. The smooth endoplasmic reticulum showed significant increases at 52 weeks in both males and females at all dietary levels. At the end of the study, notable endoplasmic reticulum increases were detected only at the highest dose levels, although non-significant increases were noted at all dose levels in both males and females. Examination of the sciatic nerve showed no effects attributable to permethrin. No oncogenic effects were noted at any dose level (Ishmael & Litchfield, 1988).

Long-Evans rats (60 males and 60 females per group) fed permethrin in the diet at dose levels of 0, 20, 100, or 500 mg/kg for 2 years did not reveal any mortality or adverse effects on growth, food consumption, or behaviour attributable to the administration. Haematology, clinical chemistry, and urinalysis measurements were performed at either 6 months or 1 year and at the end of the study. There were no compound-related effects on a wide variety of parameters examined, and ophthalmological examination indicated no abnormalities. Blood glucose levels were higher in the highest-dose males at 24 months and in the highest-dose females at 18 months, compared to the values of the control animals. Two independent evaluations of the histopathological data concluded that there was no oncogenic potential for permethrin. While there was a dose-dependent increase in gross liver weight in both males and females, these values are small and not statistically significant. The NOEL for general toxicity in this study was estimated to be 100 mg/kg (Braun & Rinehart, 1977; Billups 1978a, b).

7.6 Carcinogenesis

Summaries by Paynter et al. (1982) of toxicological data from seven long-term chronic toxicity/oncogenicity studies (four in mouse and three in rat) carried out by ICI, FMC, and Burroughs-Welcome (BW) have been made available by the US EPA. One rat study and one mouse study performed by ICI were recently published (Ishmael & Litchfield, 1988), and one rat study and one mouse study carried out by BW were cited in FAO/WHO (1988). A report of the FIFRA Scientific Advisory Panel which reviewed this data was also made available (US EPA, 1981). Table 13 summarizes the basic design of each of these studies, some of which are also discussed in section 7.5.

7.6.1 Mouse

One of the four mouse studies referenced in Table 13 (FMC I) was not considered for evaluation because of dose level changes in the mid- and high-level groups and problems in histopathological methodology.

7.6.1.1 ICI study

Relevant non-oncogenic effects observed during the study consisted of increased mortality, increased liver aminopyrine-*N*-demethylase activity, increased liver weight, and eosinophilia of hepatocytes in both males and females at 2500 mg/kg diet. The liver changes observed in this study were considered to be related in large measure to the induction of liver microsomal enzyme activity. Minimal liver changes were also observed at 1000 mg/kg, but not at 250 mg/kg. A slight increase in lung adenomas was observed in male mice at the highest dose level. However, there was some uncertainty as to whether this increase was related to permethrin ingestion.

7.6.1.2 FMC II study

Relevant non-oncogenic effects observed during the study consisted of increased mortality in males at 2000 mg/kg diet, increased liver weight in females at 2500 mg/kg and 5000 mg/kg, and increased lung weight in females at 5000 mg/kg. Histopathologically, dose-related "focal alveolar cell proliferation" (increased numbers of lung cells) was observed in permethrin-treated females. As regards oncogenic effects, there was an increased incidence of bronchio-alveolar adenomas in female mice only. The number of female mice with adenomas and/or carcinomas (15/74, 24/72, 35/74, and 44/75 at the four dose levels) revealed a statistically significant dose-response relationship. Male mice did not show this effect. However, some doubt was expressed by the FIFRA Scientific Advisory Panel concerning the conduct of this study.

7.6.1.3 BW study

Non-oncogenic effects observed during the study consisted of slightly decreased mortality in females at 50 and 250 mg/kg per day, increased liver weights in males, and increased kidney weights in females at 250 mg/kg per day. Histopathologically, an increased incidence in cuboidal/columnar metaplasia of the alveolar epithelium was observed in the lungs of male and female mice at the highest dose. The oncogenicity data indicated a dose-related trend in females, but not in males, for adenomatous tumours in the lungs. No notable pattern was observed for other neoplasms at any dose level.

7.6.1.4 Appraisal of mouse studies on carginogenicity

Consistent findings in the above three mouse studies at high dose levels were liver changes known to be associated with the induction of the liver microsomal enzyme system. Other histopathological effects observed in liver, not usually associated with microsomal induction, included multifocal hepatocytomegaly and hepatocytic pigmentation. The incidence of lung adenomas for each of the three mouse studies is given in Table 14.

Among the three long-term mouse studies, there was evidence of permethrin oncogenicity in the lungs in one strain (CD-1 female only) at the highest dose level only.

Although there was a difference between the control and treated groups in terms of lung adenomas in these studies, these differences were not significant when compared with historical control values. The oncogenicity potential, as evaluated by the FIFRA Scientific Advisory Panel, was considered to be very weak.

Table 13. Chronic toxicity and carcinogenicity studies in mice and rats

Study performed by	Species	Strain	No. of animals	Duration (weeks)	Dose (mg/kg diet)	Reference
ICI	mouse	Alderly Park (SPF)	70	98	0, 250, 1000, 2500	Ishmael & Litchfield (1988)
FMC I	mouse	CD-1	75	104	0, 20, 500, 4000	Hogan & Rinehart (1977); Rapp (1978)
FMC II	mouse	CD-1	75	104	M: 0, 20, 500, 4000 F: 0, 20, 2500, 5000	Bio Dynamics (1979)
BW	mouse	CFLP	75	92	0[a], 10[a], 50[b], 250[b]	James et al. (1980)
ICI	rat	Wistar	60	104	0, 500, 1000, 2500	Ishmael & Litchfield (1988)
FMC	rat	Long-Evans	60	104	0, 20, 100, 500	Braun & Rinehart (1977); Billups (1978a,b)
BW	rat	Wistar	60	104	0, 10[b], 50[b], 250[b]	McSheehy & Finn (1980)

a 100 animals as control.
b mg/kg body weight; permethrin 25% cis, 75% trans.

Table 14. Comparison of lung adenomas (%) in three mouse studies

	Male				Female			
	control	low dose	mid dose	high dose	control	low dose	mid dose	high dose
ICI study	20	12	26	32	22	16	20	30
FMC II study	22	23	28	25	16(20[a])	17	35	35
BW study	26	19	23	22	3(20[b])	7	10	20

a Historical control values ranged from 23 to 60%, with a mean of 20.4%.
b Historical control values ranged from 7.5 to 30.0%, with a mean of 20.4%.

7.6.2 *Rat*

One of the three long-term rat studies referred to in Table 13, i.e. the FMC rat study, was excluded from examination because of serious flaws in histopathological methodology.

7.6.2.1 *ICI study*

Relevant non-oncogenic effects observed consisted of increased mortality in males and decreased mortality in females at 2500 mg/kg diet, increased liver weights in both males and females at 1000 and 2500 mg/kg and in males only at 500 mg/kg, increased liver aminopyrine-N-demethylase activity in both males and females at 1000 and 2500 mg/kg, and hepatocyte vacuolization or hypertrophy in males and females at 1000 and 2500 mg/kg. Additional effects observed were increased kidney weight in males at all treatment levels and increased pituitary weight in males at 1000 and 2500 mg/kg.

No tumours related to the ingestion of permethrin were observed in this study.

7.6.2.2 *BW study*

Non-oncogenic effects observed at 250 mg/kg per day were increased mortality in males, occasional body tremors in males and females, increased liver weight in males, hepatocyte hypertrophy in males and females, and focal changes of the thyroid follicles in males and females. The microscopic liver and thyroid changes were also observed at 50 mg/kg per day in both sexes.

With respect to tumours (including rare, unusual, or malignant neoplasms), none of the tumour types observed in this study were considered to be related to the ingestion of permethrin.

7.6.2.3 *Appraisal of rat studies on carcinogenicity*

No evidence of oncogenicity was observed in the rat studies.

7.7 Mutagenicity

7.7.1 Microorganism and insects

The mutagenic activity of permethrin was evaluated using the Ames test. There was no increase in the number of revertant colonies at doses up to 2500 μg permethrin/plate in five strains of Salmonella typhimurium (TA1535, TA1537, TA1538, TA98, and TA100) with or without S9-mix prepared from rat liver or S9 prepared from PCB-treated mice (Longstaff, 1976; Newell & Skinner, 1976; Simmon, 1976; Suzuki, 1977).

Permethrin and six other synthetic pyrethroids were tested for mutagenicity in S. typhimurium TA98 and TA100 strains in the presence and absence of a metabolic-activation system. All pyrethroids tested gave negative results (Pluijmen et al., 1984).

Two reverse-mutation tests in *Escherichia coli* WP2 also gave negative results (Newell & Skinner, 1976; Simmon, 1976).

When tested for mutagenicity in V79 Chinese hamster cells, permethrin and five other synthetic pyrethroids were shown to be non-mutagenic (Pluijmen et al., 1984).

In a host-mediated assay, permethrin (200 mg/kg body weight) was orally administered to ICR mice. The indicator organism, S. typhimurium G46, harvested from the abdominal cavity of mice 3 h after treatment, did not reveal any mutagenic effect (Shirasu et al., 1979). In another host-mediated assay employing a similar test system, (+)-*trans*-permethrin at dose levels of 600 and 3000 mg/kg body weight and (+)-*cis*-permethrin at 21 and 54 mg/kg body weight gave negative results (Miyamoto, 1976).

Permethrin was tested for its ability to induce complete and partial chromosome loss in *Drosophila melanogaster* males by adding 5 mg/litre (soaked onto a filter paper) to the feeding solution. Treated males were mated with mus-302 repair-defective females to detect chromosome loss in the zygotes. Permethrin did not induce a significant increase in chromosome loss, compared to negative controls (Woodruff et al., 1983).

7.7.2 Mammals

An *in vivo* cytogenetic test was performed in Alderly Park rats to assess the ability of permethrin to induce chromosomal aberration. Permethrin was administered to groups of eight males by a single intraperitoneal injection or by five daily injections at doses of 600, 3000, or 6000 mg/kg. The cytogenetic effect on bone marrow cells was evaluated 24 h after the single injection and 6 h after the last multiple dosing. No differences were observed in the rate of chromosomal aberrations between any permethrin-treated groups and the vehicle controls. Two positive controls (trimethyl phosphate and mitomycin C) produced a significantly higher incidence of chromosomal aberrations (Anderson & Richardson, 1976).

Permethrin (25:75) gave a negative response when mouse lymphoma L5178Y cells were treated with permethrin (up to 125 μg/ml) with or without activation (Clive, 1977).

In dominant lethal studies, permethrin dissolved in corn oil was administered orally for five successive days to groups of male CD mice (15 per group) at doses of 15, 48, or 150 mg/kg. Each male was mated with 16 virgin females, and on the 12th day of gestation the females were killed. There was no dose-related effect on pregnancy or early or late fetal deaths. Administration of permethrin thus had no dominant lethal effect on male mice. On the other hand, the positive control (ethylmethanesulfonate) induced pre-implantation losses and the early death of embryos (McGregor & Wickramaratne, 1976a; Chesher et al., 1975b).

7.8 Teratogenicity and Reproduction Studies

7.8.1 Teratogenicity studies

7.8.1.1 Mouse

In studies by Kohda et al. (1976b), groups of pregnant ICR mice (27 to 32 mice per group) were orally administered permethrin at dose levels of 0, 15, 50, or 150 mg/kg body weight from day 7 to day 12 of pregnancy. On day 18, two-thirds of the animals were sacrificed and examined for implantation and resorption sites. Viable offspring were examined for somatic and skeletal abnormalities, and, after 3 weeks of lactation, pups were examined for behavioral abnormalities and for differentiation and growth. At 6 weeks of age, all animals were sacrificed and subjected to internal and external examination. There were no effects on maternal toxicity over the course of the study. Growth and differentiation of pregnant females were not affected by permethrin, nor were the number of implantation sites or litter size adversely affected. The size of individual pups and the incidence of gross external, internal, and skeletal abnormalities were not significantly different from those in the control mice. Permethrin, at dose levels up to and including 150 mg/kg, did not appear to affect those animals allowed to bear and wean young. The growth of young animals did not appear to differ from control values, and, 3 weeks after weaning, the surviving animals did not differ from controls with respect to growth or major organ changes. There was no teratogenicity associated with permethrin in this mouse bioassay, although the duration of dosing was a little too short to cover both the early and late stage of organ development (Kohda et al., 1976b).

7.8.1.2 Rat

In studies by McGregor & Wickramaratne (1976b), pregnant CD rats (20 rats per group) were orally administered permethrin at dose levels of 0, 22.5, 71.0, or 225 mg/kg from day 6 to day 16 of gestation. On day 20, the animals were sacrificed and the corpora lutea were examined. Somatic and skeletal investigations were performed on the fetuses. No adverse toxicological response was seen at the highest dose used. There were no abortions or maternal deaths and no significant differences in pregnancy frequency, corpora lutea, or total number of implantations between treated and control rats. Placental and fetal weights were similar to those of the controls and no skeletal or structural abnormalities were observed. Based upon the standard teratological rat bioassay, permethrin did not show any teratological potential.

Pregnant Sprague-Dawley rats (29-34 rats per group) were orally administered permethrin at dose levels of 0, 10, 20, or 50 mg/kg body weight from day 9 to day 14 of pregnancy. On day 20, approximately two-thirds of the pregnant females were sacrificed and the remaining rats were allowed to deliver and wean pups. After lactation, the pups were examined for behaviour and for growth and differentiation before being sacrificed at 6 weeks of age and examined for internal and external gross malformations. Pregnant females fed at the highest dose showed toxic signs of poisoning, including ataxia, tremor, and a slight reduction in body weight. There was no mortality, although fetal loss at the highest dose level was slightly higher than that in the control animals. A slightly higher incidence of non-ossified sternebra was noted at 50 mg/kg. The number of implantation sites and the litter size were not affected, and growth and differentiation were similarly unaffected. Internal and external examination showed that, with the exception of the slight skeletal variation noted at 50 mg/kg, there were no permethrin-associated changes. In those animals allowed to bear and wean pups, there were no notable differences from control values with respect to gestation, implantation sites, delivery, and numbers of live young. Growth and differentiation of the offspring did not appear to be affected by permethrin, and there were no abnormalities with respect to gross pathology or in the weights of major tissues and organs at the conclusion of the study. Permethrin did not elicit a teratogenic effect in this bioassay (Kohda et al., 1976a).

In a study by Metker et al. (1977), permethrin (4, 41, and 83 mg/kg/diet), aspirin (200 mg/kg diet), and corn oil (2 ml/kg diet) were each administered to groups of 20 pre-impregnated Sprague-Dawley rats from day 6 to day 16 of gestation. The animals were sacrificed on day 20 of gestation, and the fetuses were removed and examined for gross abnormalities, sex, weight, and body length. The administration of aspirin (the positive control) resulted in significantly lower body weight and length and a variety of abnormalities including craniorachioschisis in the foetuses. Permethrin, administered to pregnant rats during gestation by intragastric intubation, did not appear to present a teratogenic or lethal hazard to the developing fetus.

When groups of 22 female Wistar rats received permethrin (25:75) at 0 or 200 mg/kg body weight in corn oil by daily oral gavage on days 6-16 (inclusive) of pregnancy, treatment was without apparent effect on maternal body weight gain or general conditions. The animals were sacrificed on day 20 so that their uterine contents could be examined.

Treatment had no effect on the number of corpora lutea, implantations, live fetuses, early and late fetal deaths, or fetal abnormalities. Examination of the fetuses, which included dissection and skeletal staining, showed no morphological effects of treatment. These results indicate that permethrin (25:75) at 200 mg/kg body weight per day is not fetotoxic to rats (James, 1974).

7.8.1.3 Rabbit

Mated female Dutch rabbits (18 per group) were orally administered permethrin (at dose levels of 0, 600, 1200, or 1800 mg/kg body weight per day) in 0.5% v/v aqueous Tween 80 from days 6-18 inclusive of pregnancy. On day 29 of pregnancy the animals were killed and their uteri were examined for resorptions and live implantations. The fetuses were examined for gross abnormalities of skeleton and soft tissue. At all dose levels, permethrin depressed body weight gain during dosing and was embryotoxic at the two highest dose levels. It was toxic to the dams at 1800 mg/kg body weight per day, but no teratogenic activity was detectable at any dose level (Richards et al., 1980).

7.8.2 Reproduction Studies

7.8.2.1 Rat

Groups of Long-Evans rats (10 males and 20 females per group) were fed permethrin at dose levels of 0, 20, and 100 mg/kg diet in a 3-generation (two litters per generation) reproduction study. There was no effect on mortality, mating, pregnancy, or fertility, with the exception of the F_2 mating index, which was reduced in both controls and treatment groups. Pup survival and growth were unaffected. Haematological evaluations of F_2 adults between the second and third mating showed no unusual effects. This study indicated that dietary permethrin does not adversely affect reproduction in the rat (Schroeder & Rinehart, 1977).

In studies by Hodge et al. (1977), groups of Wistar rats (12 males and 24 females per group) were fed permethrin at dose levels of 0, 500, 1000, and 2500 mg/kg diet for 12 weeks. At 12 weeks the animals were mated to initiate a standard 3-generation (two litters per generation) reproduction study. Clinical signs of acute poisoning (tremors, etc.) were noted, predominantly in females given the highest dose. There were no effects attributable to permethrin on fertility, gestation, viability of pups, sex ratio, litter size, or lactation. Ten male and female weanlings from the second litter of the F_3 generation were examined for histopathological changes. Centrilobular hypertrophy and cytoplasmic eosinophilia were observed at all dose levels, the incidence and severity of which appeared to be dose dependent. Rats in the third litter of the F_3 generation were sacrificed on day 12 of gestation for teratogenic examination, but no abnormalities were observed. Based on the results of this study, permethrin does not appear to induce reproductive toxicity in rats.

Spencer and Berhance (1982) fed female Sprague-Dawley rats (5-8 rats per group) permethrin in the diet at levels of 0, 500, 1000, 1500, 2000, 2500, 3000, 3500, and 4000 mg/kg diet from day 6 to day 15 of pregnancy. Laparotomy was performed on day 20 of gestation, and the number of live fetuses was determined. Placentae were excised and cleaned of extraneous connective tissue. Analysis of the protein and glycogen contents of the placentae on day 16 of pregnancy indicated that they were only influenced by very high doses (2500-4000 mg/kg diet) of permethrin. Analysis of variance indicated no significant effect on protein level, but the treatment did decrease the glycogen concentration. No significant dose-related effects on implantational sites/intrauterine fetuses were observed. These results appeared to confirm that permethrin possesses low mammalian toxicity.

In a 3-generation reproduction study, groups of 20 male and 20 female Wistar COBS rats received permethrin (25:75) in the diet at 0, 5, 30, and 180 mg/kg body weight per day during growth, mating, gestation, parturition, and lactation for three generations, each with two litters. Fetal toxicity and teratogenicity was assessed in the second pregnancy of the F_2 generation. Treatment with permethrin had no effect on general behaviour or condition, food intake, body weight gain, or pregnancy rate of the dams, or on parturition, sex ratio, or pup weight. A small number of rats of each group developed eye abnormalities, including ocular haemorrhage and chronic glaucoma, but this was not related to the treatment. Examination of F_{3b} fetuses showed no treatment-related effect on sex ratio, body weight, or the occurrence of visceral or skeletal abnormalities. This study indicated that permethrin (25:75) has no effect on the reproduction of rats at doses up to 180 mg/kg body weight per day (James, 1979).

7.9 Neurotoxicity

7.9.1 Rat

When male and female Charles River rats (six of each sex per group) were fed permethrin at dose levels of 0 or 6000 mg/kg diet for up to 14 days, severe clinical signs of poisoning were evident in all the permethrin-treated rats. Only one permethrin-treated male survived the 14-day trial. Fragmented and swollen sciatic nerve axons and myelin degeneration were observed in four out of five permethrin-treated animals (Hend & Butterworth, 1977).

In a short-term study designed to assess the effects of high concentrations of permethrin on the sciatic nerve, male Wistar rats (10 per group) were fed permethrin at dose levels of 0, 2500, 3000, 3750, 4500, 5000, and 7000 mg/kg diet for 14 days. Clinical signs of acute poisoning and death occurred in the animals that were dosed at 5000 or 7000 mg/kg. Some rats that received the lower dose levels showed slight to moderate tremors, and food consumption and growth were reduced in these animals. At the two lowest dose levels, clinical signs of poisoning disappeared within the first week whereas, at the higher dose levels, signs of poisoning persisted throughout the study. Rats receiving permethrin at doses of up to 4500 mg/kg showed no ultra-structural changes in their sciatic nerve. A variety of mild ultra-structural changes, such as vacuolation and swelling of unmyelinated fibres and hypertrophy of Schwann cells, were observed in the nerves of rats receiving 5000 mg/kg (Glaister et al., 1977).

A detailed morphological evaluation of the nervous system was performed on rats in two long-term feeding studies. In the first, Long-Evans rats were fed diets containing permethrin at concentrations of 0, 20, 100, or 500 mg/kg diet for 2 years, and five male and five female randomly selected survivors from each group were examined. In the second study, Long-Evans rats were fed diets containing permethrin at concentrations of 0, 20, or 100 mg/kg diet for three successive generations, and five male and five female rats from each group were randomly selected from the third generation parental animals. Examination of central and peripheral nerves and of extensive morphometric data and teased myelinated fibers of distal sural and tibial nerves and of the maxillary division of the fifth cranial nerve did not reveal any changes attributable to the feeding of the pesticide (Dyck et al., 1984).

When groups of 10 male and 10 female Sprague-Dawley rats were given permethrin (25:75) (94.5% pure) at 4000, 6000, or 9000 mk/kg diet for 21 days, all animals developed severe trembling and lost weight. Some of the highest-dose rats of each sex died. Subsequent examination of brain, spinal cord, trigeminal and dorsal root ganglia, proximal and distal root trunks, and terminal motor and sensory nerves revealed no consistent histopathological abnormalities (Dayan, 1980).

7.9.2 Hen

Hens were administered permethrin orally (cis:trans=1:1) (as a 40% w/v solution in dimethylsulfoxide) at a daily dose level of 1 g/kg body weight for 5 days. After 3 weeks, the dosing regimen was repeated, and the animals were maintained for an additional period of 3 weeks before being sacrificed. There were no signs of neurological disturbance or mortality in any of the animals. All hens treated with tri-*ortho*-cresyl phosphate (TOCP) (positive control) displayed clinical and histopathological evidence of neurotoxicity, whereas none of the birds dosed with permethrin showed any signs of intoxication. Histological examination of nerve tissues revealed no lesions. Hence, permethrin was considered to have no delayed neurotoxic potential such as that associated with certain organophosphates (Millner & Butterworth, 1977).

In studies by Ross & Prentice (1977), 15 adult hens were orally administered permethrin at 9 g/kg body weight and again 21 days later. After a further 21 days, they were sacrificed. All positive control animals (given TOCP at 500 mg/kg) showed signs of delayed neurotoxicity ranging from slight muscular incoordination to paralysis. No signs of ataxia were recorded in any of the hens in the permethrin-treated or negative control groups. Histopathological examination of the nervous tissues of permethrin-treated animals revealed none of the degenerative changes noted in the tissues of the positive controls.

7.10 Behavioural Effects

Behavioural observations were carried out on immature male Sprague-Dawley rats habituated to inhalation of permethrin aerosols. Habituation was carried out by exposing three groups of rats (five per group) to aerosols of permethrin firstly at 500 mg/m^3 for 21 days, then at 1000 mg/m^3 for an additional 21 days. Three other groups of rats (five per group) served as controls; they were similarly treated but were not exposed to permethrin. At the end of this conditioning period, all rats, including the controls, were exposed to a permethrin aerosol at 5000 mg/m^3 for 4 h. At the end of the habituation period, there were no differences in retention of avoidance training or the ability to learn the same task between controls and aerosol-exposed groups. However, after exposure to permethrin at 5000 mg/m^3, the non-habituated control group of rats showed significantly lower retention capacity compared with the habituated rats or with their own pre-exposure performances. The non-habituated control rats also showed decreases in coordination and balance and a higher incidence of conflict behaviour and tremors. The performance of the rats in the habituated groups was not changed (Sherman, 1979).

7.11 Miscellaneous Studies

The pharmacological action of permethrin on nictitating membrane, blood pressure, respiration, heart rate, and isolated ileum was investigated in the rabbit, guinea-pig, and cat. Permethrin reduced the incidence and amplitude of contraction of isolated rabbit ileum but induced no changes in a similar preparation from the guinea-pig. Intravenous administration of permethrin at doses of 4 mg/kg or more affected blood pressure and respiration in all animals. The hypotensive effect was not affected by pretreatment with atropine or propanolol. Permethrin was shown to produce slight contraction of the nictitating membrane. An increase in pulse rate was observed in the electrocardiogram (ECG) of the rabbit at dose levels above 4 mg/kg, but was not accompanied by changes in the wave pattern (Nomura & Segawa, 1979).

In the Japanese White rabbit, the intravenous administration of lethal doses of permethrin caused changes in the electroencephalogram (EEG) tracings. Spike waves and an increased amplitude of slow waves were induced at 100 mg/kg body weight. At a sub-lethal dose of 30 mg/kg, permethrin did not induce changes in the EEG (Takahashi et al., 1979).

There was no change in hexobarbital-induced sleeping time in ICR mice intraperitoneously administered a single dose of permethrin at dose levels of up to 2000 mg/kg body weight (Takahashi et al., 1979).

Sprague-Dawley rats (three groups of 10 rats each) were pretreated for four consecutive days with an intraperitoneal injection of either sodium phenobarbital at 100 mg/kg (positive control group), permethrin at 575 mg/kg (test group), or corn oil at 2.0 ml/kg (solvent control group). On the fifth test day the rats received an intraperitoneal injection of hexobarbital (220 mg/kg). The hexobarbital-induced sleeping times of the permethrin-treated rats were significantly shorter than those of the solvent control animals but were similar to those of the phenobarbital positive control (Metker et al., 1977).

Permethrin and cypermethrin were evaluated for their ability to alter microsomal cytochrome P-450 and NADPH cytochrome *c* reductase in Long-Evans rats. When permethrin (cis:trans = 80:20) was orally administered to rats at 50 mg/kg body weight per day, it increased cytochrome P-450 after 4, 8, or 12 days of administration and NADPH cytochrome *c* reductase after 8 or 12 days, whereas cypermethrin (α-cyano analogue of permethrin) did not induce either cytochrome P-450 or the reductase. Neither of the two pyrethroids altered body weight gain (Carlson & Schoening, 1980).

7.12 Mechanism of Toxicity (Mode of Action)

Based on the signs of toxicity to mammals (Verschoyle & Aldridge, 1980; Lawrence & Casida, 1982) and to cockroaches (Gammon et al., 1981), pyrethroids may be classified into two types: Type I and Type II compounds (see Appendix I). 1R-*cis*- and 1R-*trans*-permethrin belong to Type I. Electrophysiological recordings from dosed cockroaches reveal trains of cercal sensory spikes and, sometimes, spike trains from the cercal motor nerves and the central nervous system. The signs of poisoning caused by Type I pyrethroid compounds are restlessness, incoordination, hyperactivity, prostration, and paralysis (Gammon et al., 1981).

1RS-*cis*-permethrin and 1RS-*trans*-permethrin cause tremor (known as T-syndrome) when injected intravenously into rats at a dose level of more than 270 mg/kg body weight. The onset of the T-syndrome is usually rapid. Rats suffering from T-syndrome exhibit aggressive sparring behaviour and increased sensitivity to external stimuli. This is followed by the appearance of a slight tremor, which gradually becomes more severe and finally reaches a state of prostration and vigorous whole body tremor. The core temperature is markedly increased during poisoning; this may result from the excessive muscular activity associated with tremor (Verschoyle & Aldridge, 1980).

Exposure of sensory nerve fibres from clawed frogs (*Xenopus laevis*) to permethrin (10^{-7} to 10^{-5} mol/litre) resulted in marked repetitive activity. This heightened activity was not observed in the motor fibres of frogs that were similarly tested. Treatment of isolated lateral-line preparations of frogs with permethrin (5×10^{-6} mol/litre) also resulted in pronounced repetitive activity (Van den Bercken & Vijverberg, 1980b).

Permethrin (cis, trans, and technical grade) and deltamethrin, as representatives of the non-cyano- and cyano-containing classes, respectively, of synthetic pyrethroids, were examined regarding their major site of action on the mammalian nervous system in mice. ED_{50} values for the ability of both types of pyrethroids to cause prostration and loss of righting reflex were estimated following either intravenous or intracerebroventricular injections. The comparative potencies of the four pyrethroids (deltamethrin > *cis*-permethrin > technical grade permethrin > *trans*-permethrin) were the same following either route of administration. All four compounds tested showed a much greater potency (> 200-fold for deltamethrin, *cis*-permethrin, and technical grade permethrin, and 85-fold for *trans*-permethrin) after intracerebroventricular administration than after intravenous administration. In addition, the poisoning symptoms seen following direct central injection were almost identical to those obtained with peripheral administration. These results suggest that poisoning from both classes of pyrethroids in mammals is due predominantly to central mechanisms (Staatz et al., 1982).

8. EFFECTS ON HUMANS

Although permethrin has been used for many years, no human poisoning cases have been reported.

8.1 Occupational Exposure

Data on permethrin human toxicity are scanty. Studies of occupational exposure to permethrin were reported in Sweden (Kolmodin-Hedman et al., 1982). In the first study, six forestry workers using an aqueous emulsion of permethrin (trans:cis=75:25) were studied. The duties of these workers involved dipping conifer seedlings in a 2% aqueous emulsion of permethrin (one worker) and packaging the permethrin-treated seedlings (five workers). The permethrin concentrations in the breathing zones of these workers varied between 0.011 and 0.085 mg/m^3. One person excreted permethrin metabolites at 0.26 μg/ml urine the following morning, but the same afternoon the urinary excretion of permethrin residues was below the detection limit of 0.1 μg/ml. The urine from other workers did not contain detectable amounts of permethrin residues. No symptoms of permethrin poisoning were reported in this field study. The second study, performed on the basis of a questionnaire and interviews, was conducted 1-2 months after the planting season. It involved 87 persons at various plant nurseries that used the insecticide (trans:cis=60:40 or 75/25). This study showed that the major work-related symptoms amongst workers were irritative, such as itching and burning of the skin, and itching and irritation of the eyes. Irritative symptoms in the skin and upper respiratory tract were reported in 63% of workers who were exposed to permethrin (trans:cis=75:25) and 33% who were exposed to permethrin with a different isomeric composition (trans:cis=60:40). The frequency of each symptom was about 10% in each case. Increased nasal secretion was reported by 13% of the workers handling permethrin (trans:cis= 75:25).

Le Quesne et al. (1980) examined 23 laboratory workers involved in field trials, formulation, or general laboratory work with permethrin, cypermethrin, fenvalerate, and fenpropathrin. The study involved electrophysiological monitoring and interviews to ascertain subjective symptoms. The most frequently reported symptom was a facial sensation described as tingling, burning, or nettle rash by workers who had experienced it on one or more occasions. This sensation usually occurred about 30 min to 3 h after exposure and lasted for about 30 min to 8 h. Apparently this did not occur when permethrin alone was involved. All the workers were examined neurologically and no abnormal findings were recorded. Electro-physiological measurements from these workers were compared with those of an age-matched control group. No difference in response was found between the two groups.

Studies of pesticide contamination of clothing worn by crop consultants during permethrin application to soybean fields were performed to assess the extent of dermal exposure to the pesticide. The suits and T-shirts were removed and wrapped in aluminum foil, placed on ice and transported to the laboratory where they were held in a freezer until residue analysis was performed. Specimens from the thigh, arm, and chest of each suit and from the arm and chest of each T-shirt were collected, extracted with hexane and analyzed by GC-ECD. Measurable residues of permethrin were detected only in leg specimens (Cloud et al., 1987).

As part of an evaluation of permethrin (25:75) (5% wettable powder) in Nigeria, medical surveillance, including urinalysis of staff engaged in bagging, mixing, or spraying, was undertaken. Medical history, pulse, and blood pressure were recorded and urine was collected twice daily. This surveillance revealed no effects attributable to permethrin. Despite the use of protective clothing, up to 2 mg of permethrin was excreted within 24 h of exposure (Rishikesh et al., 1978).

8.2 Clinical Studies

Flannigan & Tucker (1985) and Flannigan et al. (1985a,b) studied the difference in the degree of paraesthesia induced by a number of pyrethroids. On five occasions, 0.05 ml of field-strength-formulated permethrin (0.13 mg/cm^2) was applied to a 4 cm^2 area of earlobe. The opposite earlobe received distilled water. Participant evaluation after each application continued for 48 h and involved description of the cutaneous sensations. Each participant was treated after each application with one of the remaining compounds. Permethrin, like the other pyrethroids, induced skin sensations. Paraesthesia developed with a latency period of approximately 30 min, peaked by 8 h, and deteriorated within 24 h. In the case of permethrin these sensations were approximately four times less marked than those induced by cypermethrin and fenvalerate, which both contain an α-cyano-group. It was also found that local application of dl-α-tocopheryl acetate markedly inhibited the occurrence of skin sensations.

To assess the safety of permethrin dusts for the control of human body lice, approximately 350 people were individually dusted with 50 g of powder containing either 2.5 or 5.0 g permethrin/kg. Urine samples, taken at the time of treatment and subsequently, indicated that maximal absorption of permethrin was 39 μg/kg, 24 h after treatment (Nassif et al., 1980).

In a study to assess the degree of dermal absorption of permethrin from impregnated clothing, a group of 10 male volunteer soldiers for 48 h wore military clothing that had previously been treated with an aqueous suspension of permethrin (0.2% w/v). Subsequent analysis showed that the mean permethrin (25:75) concentration of the shirts and trousers was 0.32 g/100 g. However, the average individual exposure to permethrin was 3.8 mg/day. No volunteers complained of irritation and there were no abnormal findings on physical examination (Farquhar et al., 1981a).

When dermally exposed to permethrin [(25:75) 1% w/w in soft paraffin] for up to 9 days using a patch test, 2 out of 17 volunteers developed mild erythema (Pegum & Doughty, 1978).

To assess the human tolerance, absorption, and persistence of permethrin when used against human lice, 10 adult volunteers (four men, six women) were treated with 15-40 ml of permethrin (25:75) (1%) head louse solution. Their hair was allowed to dry naturally and then washed with baby shampoo. Urine samples were collected at 0-24, 24-48, 120-144, and 336-360 h to measure dermal absorption. On assessment, 3 out of 10 volunteers developed mild, patchy erythema, which faded between days 4-7. Permethrin excretion during the first 24 h was only about 1% of the applied dose, while the cumulative maximum over 14 days was only about 5.5 mg (Farquhar et al., 1981b).

9. PREVIOUS EVALUATIONS BY INTERNATIONAL BODIES

The Joint FAO/WHO Meeting on Pesticide Residues (JMPR) discussed and evaluated permethrin in 1979, 1980, 1981, 1982, 1983, 1984, 1985, and 1987 (FAO/WHO, 1980a,b; 1981a,b; 1982a,b; 1983a,b; 1984a,b; 1985a,b; 1986a,b; 1987).

An acceptable daily intake (ADI) of 0-0.05 mg/kg body weight (cis:trans ratios of 40:60 and 27:75) was established in 1985.

Maximum residue limits of 0.01-50 mg/kg for specified foods and 20-100 mg/kg dry weight for specified feed have been proposed (FAO/WHO, 1986).

In the WHO recommended classification of pesticides by hazard, permethrin as a technical product is classified in class II (i.e. as moderately hazardous) (WHO, 1988). A WHO/FAO data sheet on permethrin exists (WHO/FAO, 1984).

REFERENCES

AGNIHOTRI, N.P., JAIN, H.K., & GAJBHIYE, V.T. (1986) Persistence of some synthetic pyrethroid insecticides in soil, water and sediment - Part I. *J. entomol. Res.*, **10**: 147-151.

ALINIAZEE, M.T. & CRANHAM, J.E. (1980) Effect of four synthetic pyrethroids on a predatory mite, *Typhlodromus pyri*, and its prey, *Panonychus ulmi*, on apples in southeast England. *Environ. Entomol.*, **9**: 436-439.

ANDERSON, D. & RICHARDSON, C.R. (1976) *Permethrin (PP557): cytogenetic study in the rat* (Report No. CTL/P/296) (Unpublished report submitted to WHO by ICI Central Toxicology Laboratory).

ANDERSON, R.L. (1982) Toxicity of fenvalerate and permethrin to several nontarget aquatic invertebrates. *Environ. Entomol.*, **11**: 1251-1257.

BAKER, P.G. & BOTTOMLEY, P. (1982) Determination of residues of synthetic pyrethroids in fruit and vegetables by gas-liquid and high-performance liquid chromatography. *Analyst*, **107**: 206-212.

BATTELLE (1982) *Pesticide programme of research and market planning. Part I: Insecticides*, Geneva, Institut Battelle (October 1982).

BATTELLE (1986) *World Pesticide Programme, Insecticide II, 1984*, Geneva, Institut Battelle.

BILLUPS, L.H. (1978a) *Histopathologic examination of a twenty-four month toxicity/carcinogenicity study of compound FMC33297 in rats*, (Unpublished report submitted to WHO by FMC Corporation, Environmental Pathology Services).

BILLUPS, L.H. (1978b) *Twenty-four month toxicity/carcinogenicity study of compound FMC33297 in rats* (Unpublished report submitted to WHO by FMC Corporation, Environmental Pathology Services).

BIO-DYNAMICS (1979) *Twenty-four month toxicity/carcinogenicity study of permethrin in mice* (Bio-Dynamics Inc. Project No. 76-1695/9) (Unpublished report submitted to WHO by FMC Corporation).

BORTHWICH, P.W. & WALSH, G.E. (1981) *Initial toxicological assessment of Ambush, Bolero, Bux, Dursban, Fentrifanil, Larvin, and Pydrin: Static acute toxicity tests with selected estuarine algae, invertebrates, and fish*, Springfield, Virginia, National Technical Information Service, pp. 1-9 (EPA-600/4-81-076).

BRADBROOK, C., BANHAM, P.B., GORE, C.W., PRATT, I., & WEIGHT, T.M. (1977) *PP557: A study of the reversibility of hepatic biochemical and ultrastructural changes in the rat* (Report No. CTL/P/354) (Unpublished Data submitted to WHO by ICI Central Toxicology Laboratory).

BRAUN, W.G. & KILLEEN, J.C. (1975) *Acute oral toxicity in rat: compound no. FMC33297* (Bio-Dynamics Inc. Project) (Unpublished report submitted to WHO by FMC Corporation).

BRAUN, W.G. & RINEHART, W.E. (1977) *A twenty-four month oral toxicity/carcinogenicity study of FMC33297 in rats* (Bio-Dynamics Inc. Project) (Unpublished report submitted to WHO by FMC Corporation).

BRAUN, H.E. & STANEK, J. (1982) Application of the AOAC multi-residue method to determination of synthetic pyrethroid residues in celery and animal products. *J. Assoc. Off. Anal. Chem.*, **65**: 685-689.

BUTTERWORTH, S.T.G. & HEND, R.W. (1976) *Toxicity studies on the insecticide WL43470: a five week feeding study in rats* (Report No. TLGR.0056.76) (Unpublished data submitted to WHO by Shell Research Ltd).

CARLSON, G.P. & SCHOENIG, G.P. (1980) Induction of liver microsomal NADPH cytochrome c reductase and cytochrome P-450 by some new synthetic pyrethroids. *Toxicol. appl. Pharmacol.*, **52**: 507-512.

CARROLL, B.R., WILLIS, G.H., & GRAVES, J.B. (1981) Permethrin concentration of cotton plants, persistence in soil and loss in runoff. *J. environ. Qual.*,**10**: 497-500.

CHESHER, B.C. & MALONE, J.C. (1974a) *10-day cumulative oral toxicity study with 21Z73 in rabbits*, Berkhamsted, Wellcome Research Laboratories (Report No. HEFG 74-7) (Unpublished data submitted to WHO).

CHESHER, B.C. & MALONE, J.C. (1974b) *Guinea pig sensitization study with 21Z73 using the maximisation test method*, Berkhamsted, Wellcome Research Laboratories (Report No. HEFG 74-3) (Unpublished data submitted to WHO).

CHESHER, B.C. & MALONE, J.C. (1974c) *Occular irritancy of 21Z73 in rabbits*, Berkhamsted, Wellcome Research Laboratories (Report no. HEFG 74-6) (Unpublished data submitted to WHO).

CHESHER, B.C., CLAMPITT, R.C., & MALONE, J.C. (1975) *21Z73 - Preliminary investigations into the cumulative oral toxicity on dogs*, Berkhamsted, Wellcome Research Laboratories (Report no. HEFG 75-9) (Unpublished data submitted to WHO).

CLAPP, M.J.L., BANHAM, P.B., CHART, I.S., GLAISTER, J., GORE, C., & MOYES, A. (1977a) *PP557: 28 day feeding study in rats* (Report No. CTL/P/355) (Unpublished data submitted to WHO by ICI Central Toxicology Laboratory).

CLAPP, M.J.L., BANHAM, P.B., GLAISTER, J.R., & MOYES, A. (1977b) *PP557: 28 day feeding study in mice* (Report No. CTL/P/354) (Unpublished data submitted to WHO by ICI Central Toxicology Laboratory).

CLARK, D.G. (1978) *Toxicology of WL 43479: acute toxicity of WL43479*, Sittingbourne, Shell Research Ltd (Report No. TLGR. 0043.78) (Unpublished data submitted to WHO).

CLIVE, C.D. (1977) *Mutagenicity of BW21Z73 in L5178Y/TK mouse lymphoma cells with and without exogenous metabolic activation*, Research Triangle Park, NC, Burroughs Wellcome Co. (Report No. TTEP/77/0011) (Unpublished data submitted to WHO).

CLOUD, R.M., ZIMPFER, M.L., YANES, J.JR., BOETHEL, D.J., BUCO, P., & HARMON, C.W. (1987) Insecticide residues on clothing worn by crop consultants in soybean fields treated with non-conventional application technology. *Bull. environ. Contam. Toxicol.*, **38**: 277-282.

COATS, J.R. & O'DONNELL-JEFFERY, N.L. (1979) Toxicity of four synthetic pyrethroid insecticides to rainbow trout. *Bull. environ. Contam. Toxicol.*, **23**: 250-255.

COX, R.L. & WILSON, W.T. (1984) Effects of permethrin on the behavior of individually tagged honey bees, *Apis mellifera L.* (Hymenoptera: Apidae). *Environ. Entomol.*, **13**: 375-378.

CRIDLAND, J.S. & WEATHERLEY, B.C. (1977a) *Urinary excretion in man of 3-(2,2-dichlorovinyl)-2,2-dimethylcyclopropane carboxylic acid ("CVA") after oral ingestion of permethrin (NRDC 143) - A first report*, Bechenham, Wellcome Research Laboratories (Report No. BDPE-77-1) (Unpublished data submitted to WHO).

CRIDLAND, J.S. & WEATHERLEY, B.C. (1977b) *An estimate of permethrin (NRDC 143; OMS1821) absorbed by people employed in a field trial of the insecticide*, Bechenham, Wellcome Research Laboratories (Report No. BDPE-77-3) (Unpublished data submitted to WHO).

DAYAN, A.D. (1980) 21-day neuropathological study in the Sprague-Dawley rat of permethrin (212732J) administered in the diet, Berkhamsted, Wellcome Research Laboratories (Report No. BP 80-48) (Unpublished report submitted to WHO by Wellcome Foundation Ltd).

DOYLE, R.D., KAUFMAN, D.D., BURT, G.W., & DOUGLASS, L. (1981) Degradation of *cis*-permethrin in soil amended with sewage sludge or dairy manure. *J. agric. food Chem.*, **29**: 412-414.

DYCK, P.J., SHIMONO, M., SCHOENING, G.P., LAIS, A.C., OVIATT, K.F., & SPARKS, M.F. (1984) The evaluation of a new synthetic pyrethroid pesticide (permethrin) for neurotoxicity. *J. environ. Pathol. Toxicol. Oncol.*, **5**: 109-117.

EDWARDS, D.B., OSBORN, B.E., DENT, N.J., & KINCH, D.A. (1976) *Toxicity study in beagle dogs (oral administration for three months)*, Inveresk, United Kingdom, Inveresk Research International Ltd (Submitted to WHO by ICI Ltd).

EDWARDS, M.J. & ISWARAN, T.J. (1977) *Permethrin: residue transfer and toxicology study with cows fed treated grass nuts* (Report No. TMJ1519/B) (Unpublished report submitted to WHO by ICI Plant Protection Division).

ELLIOTT, M. (1977) *Synthetic pyrethroids*, Washington, DC, American Chemical Society, p. 229 (ACS Symposium Series 42).

ELLIOTT, M., FARNHAM, A.W., JANES, N.F., NEEDHAM, P.H., PULMAN, D.A., & STEVENSON, J.H. (1973) A photostable pyrethroid. *Nature (Lond.)*, **246**: 169-170.

ELLIOTT, M., JANES, N.F., PULMAN, D.A., GAUGHAN, L.C., UNAI, T., & CASIDA, J.E. (1976) Radiosynthesis and metabolism in rats of the 1R-isomers of the insecticide permethrin. *J. agric. food Chem.*, **24**: 270-276.

EVANS, M.H. (1976) End-plate potentials in frog muscle exposed to a synthetic pyrethroid *Pestic. Biochem. Physiol.*, **6**: 547-550.

EVERTS, J.W., KORTENHOFF, B.A., HOOGLAND, H., VLUG, H.J., JOCQUE, R., & KOEMAN, J.H. (1985) Effects on non-target terrestrial arthropods of synthetic pyrethroids used for the control of the tsetse fly (*Glossina* spp.) in settlement areas of the southern Ivory Coast, Africa. *Arch. environ. Contam. Toxicol.*, **14**: 641-650.

FAO (1982) *Second Government Consultation on International Harmonization of Pesticide Registration Requirements, Rome, 11-15 October 1982*, Rome, Food and Agriculture Organization of the United Nations.

FAO/WHO (1980a) *Pesticide residues in food. Report of the 1979 Joint Meeting of the FAO Panel of Experts on Pesticide Residues in Food and the Environment and the WHO Expert Group on Pesticide Residues*, Rome, Food and Agriculture Organization of the United Nations, pp. 52-55 (FAO Plant Production and Protection Paper 20).

FAO/WHO (1980b) *1979 Evaluations of some pesticide residues in food*, Rome, Food and Agriculture Organization of the United Nations, pp. 369- 425 (FAO Plant Production and Protection Paper 20 Sup).

FAO/WHO (1981a) *Pesticide residues in food. Report of the 1980 Joint Meeting of the FAO Panel of Experts on Pesticide Residues in Food and the Environment and the WHO Expert Group on Pesticide Residues*, Rome, Food and Agriculture Organization of the United Nations, pp. 50-51 (FAO Plant Production and Protection Paper 26).

FAO/WHO (1981b) *1980 Evaluations of some pesticide residues in food*, Rome, Food and Agriculture Organization of the United Nations, pp. 360-393 (FAO Plant Production and Protection Paper 26 Sup).

FAO/WHO (1982a) *Pesticide residues in food. Report of the 1981 Joint Meeting of the FAO Panel of Experts on Pesticide Residues in Food and the Environment and the WHO Expert Group on Pesticide Residues*, Rome, Food and Agriculture Organization of the United Nations, pp. 37-39 (FAO Plant Production and Protection Paper 37).

FAO/WHO (1982b) *1981 Evaluations of some pesticide residues in food*, Rome, Food and Agriculture Organization of the United Nations, pp. 385-425 (FAO Plant Production and Protection Paper 42).

FAO/WHO (1983a) *Pesticide residues in food. Report of the 1982 Joint Meeting of the FAO Panel of Experts on Pesticide Residues in Food and the Environment and the WHO Expert Group on Pesticide Residues*, Rome, Food and Agriculture Organization of the United Nations, pp. 36-38 (FAO Plant Production and Protection Paper 46).

FAO/WHO (1983b) *1982 Evaluations of some pesticide residues in food*, Rome, Food and Agriculture Organization of the United Nations, pp. 329-350 (FAO Plant Production and Protection Paper 49).

FAO/WHO (1984a) *Pesticide residues in food. Report of the 1983 Joint Meeting of the FAO Panel of Experts on Pesticide Residues in Food and the Environment and the WHO Expert Group on Pesticide Residues*, Rome, Food and Agriculture Organization of the United Nations, p. 38, 57, 62, 65 (FAO Plant Production and Protection Paper 56).

FAO/WHO (1984b) *1983 Evaluations of some pesticide residues in food*, Rome, Food and Agriculture Organization of the United Nations, pp. 307-313, 501 (FAO Plant Production and Protection Paper 61).

FAO/WHO (1985a) *Pesticide residues in food. Report of the 1984 Joint Meeting of the FAO Panel of Experts on Pesticide Residues in Food and the Environment and the WHO Expert Group on Pesticide Residues*, Rome, Food and Agriculture Organization of the United Nations, pp. 63, 85, 93 (FAO Plant Production and Protection Paper 62).

FAO/WHO (1985b) *1984 Evaluations of some pesticide residues in food,* Rome, Food and Agriculture Organization of the United Nations, pp. 441-444, 723 (FAO Plant Production and Protection Paper 67).

FAO/WHO (1985c) *Guide to Codex recommendations concerning pesticide residues. Part 8. Recommendations for methods of analysis of pesticide residues,* 3rd ed., Rome, Codex Committee on Pesticide Residues.

FAO/WHO (1986a) *Pesticide residues in food. Report of the 1985 Joint Meeting of the FAO Panel of Experts on Pesticide Residues in Food and the Environment and the WHO Expert Group on Pesticide Residues,* Rome, Food and Agriculture Organization of the United Nations, p. 37 (FAO Plant Production and Protection Paper 68).

FAO/WHO (1986b) *1985 Evaluations of some pesticide residues in food, Part I - Residues,* Rome, Food and Agriculture Organization of the United Nations, pp. 201-203 (FAO Plant Production and Protection Paper No 72/1).

FAO/WHO (1986c) *Codex Maximum Limits for pesticide residues,* 2nd ed., Rome, Food and Agriculture Organization of the United Nations, Joint FAO/WHO Food Standards Programme, Codex Alimentarius Commission, (CAC XIII).

FAO/WHO (1987) *Pesticide residues in food. Report of the 1987 Joint Meeting of the FAO Panel of Experts on Pesticide residues in Food and the Environment and the WHO Expert Group on Pesticide Residues,* Rome, Food and Agriculture Organization of the United Nations, p. 33 (FAO Plant Production and Protection Paper 84).

FAO/WHO (1988) Permethrin. In: *Pesticide residues in food. Part II - Toxicology,* Rome, Food and Agriculture Organization of the United Nations, pp. 101-110 (FAO Plant Production and Protection Paper 86/2).

FARQUHAR, J.A., HUTCHINSON, D.B.A., PERIAM, A.W., & SPARKES, R.G. (1981a) *An investigation into the absorption of permethrin from impregnated clothing,* Bechenham, Wellcome Research Laboratories (Report No. BKDL/81/1) (Unpublished data submitted to WHO).

FARQUHAR, J.A., HUTCHINSON, D.B.A., PERIAM, A.W., & SPARKES, R.G. (1981b) *An investigation of tolerance to absorption of and persistence of permethrin applied as a 1% lotion to human hair,* Bechenham, Wellcome Research Laboratories (Report No. BKDL/81/2) (Unpublished data submitted to WHO).

FLANNIGAN, S.A. & TUCKER, S.B. (1985) Variation in cutaneous sensation between synthetic pyrethroid insecticides. *Contact Dermatitis*, **13**: 140-147.

FLANNIGAN, S.A., TUCKER, S.B., MARCUS, M.K., ROSS, C.E., FAIRCHILD, E.J., GRIMES, B.A., & HARRIST, R.B. (1985a) Primary irritant contact dermatitis from synthetic pyrethroid insecticide exposure. *Arch. Toxicol.*, **56**, 288-294.

FLANNIGAN, S.A., TUCKER, S.B., KEY, M.M., ROSS, C.E., FAIRCHILD, E.J., GRIMES, B.A., & HARRIST, R.B. (1985b) Synthetic pyrethroid insecticides: a dermatological evaluation. *Br. J. ind. Med.*, **42**: 363-372.

FRIESEN, M.K., GALLOWAY, T.D., & FLANNAGAN, J.F. (1983) Toxicity of the insecticide permethrin in water and sediment to nymphs of the burrowing mayfly *Hexagenia rigida* (Ephemeroptera: Ephemeridae). *Can. Entomol.*, 115: 1007-1014.

GAMBRELL, R.P., REDDY, C.N., COLLARD, V., GREEN, G., & PATRICK, W.H., Jr. (1981) *Behavior of DDT, kepone and permethrin in sediment-water systems under different oxidation-reduction and pH conditions*, Washington, DC, US Environmental Protection Agency (EPA 600/3-81-038).

GAMMON, D.W. & CASIDA, J.E. (1983) Pyrethroids of the most potent class antagonize GABA action at the crayfish neuromuscular junction. *Neurosci. Lett.*, **40**: 163-168.

GAMMON, D.W., BROWN, M.A., & CASIDA, J.E. (1981) Two classes of pyrethroid action in the cockroach. *Pestic. Biochem. Physiol.*, **15**: 181-191.

GAMMON, D.W., LAWRENCE, L.J., & CASIDA, J.E. (1982) Pyrethroid toxicology: Protective effects of Diazepam and phenobarbital in the mouse and the cockroach. *Toxicol. appl. Pharmacol.*, **66**: 290-296.

GAUGHAN, L.C. & CASIDA, J.E. (1978) Degradation of *trans*- and *cis*-permethrin on cotton and bean plants. *J. agric. food Chem.*, **26**: 525-528.

GAUGHAN, L.C., UNAI, T., & CASIDA, J.E. (1977) Permethrin metabolism in rats. *J. agric. food Chem.*, **25**: 9-17.

GAUGHAN, L.C., ROBINSON, R.A., & CASIDA, J.E. (1978b) Distribution and metabolic fate of *trans*- and *cis*-permethrin in laying hens. *J. agric. food Chem.*, **26**: 1374-1380.

GAUGHAN, L.C., ACKERMAN, M.E., UNAI, T., & CASIDA, J.E. (1978a) Distribution and metabolism of *trans*- and *cis*-permethrin in lactating Jersey cows. *J. agric. food Chem.*, **26**: 613-618.

GERIG, L. (1985) Testing the toxicity of synthetic pyrethroid insecticides to bees. *Pestic. Sci.*, **16**: 206-207.

GLAISTER, J.R., PRATT, I., & RICHARDS, D. (1977) *Effects of high dietary levels of PP557 on clinical behaviour and structure of sciatic nerves in rats* (Report No. CTL/P/317) (Unpublished data submitted to WHO by ICI Central Toxicology Laboratory).

GLICKMAN, A.H. & CASIDA, J.E. (1982) Species and structural variations affecting pyrethroid neurotoxicity. *Neurobehav. Toxicol. Teratol.*, **4**: (6) 793-799.

GLICKMAN, A.H. & LECH, J.J. (1981) Hydrolysis of permethrin, a pyrethroid insecticide, by rainbow trout and mouse tissues *in vitro:* A comparative study. *Toxicol. appl. Pharmacol.*, **60**: 186-192.

GLICKMAN, A.H., SHONO, T., CASIDA, J.E., & LECH, J.J. (1979) *In vitro* metabolism of permethrin isomers by carp and rainbow trout liver microsomes. *J. agric. food Chem.*, **27**: 1038-1041.

GLICKMAN, A.H., HAMID, A.AR., RICKERT, D.E., & LECH, J.J. (1981) Elimination and metabolism of permethrin isomers in rainbow trout. *Toxicol. appl. Pharmacol.*, **57**: 88-98.

GLICKMAN, A.H., WEITMAN, S.D., & LECH, J.J. (1982) Different toxicity of *trans*-permethrin in rainbow trout and mice. I. Role of biotransformation. *Toxicol. appl. Pharmacol.*, **66**: 153-161.

HAGLEY, E.A.C., PREE, D.J., & HOLLIDAY, N.J. (1980) Toxicity of insecticides to some orchard carabids (*Coleoptera carabidae*). *Can. Entomol.*, **112**: 457-462.

HALLS, G.R.H. (1981) *The fate of permethrin residues on wheat during 9 months storage in Australia* (Report No. HEFH 81-1) (Unpublished data submitted to WHO by Wellcome Research Laboratories).

HALLS, G.R.H. & PERIAM, A.W. (1980) *The fate of permethrin residues on wheat during storage and after milling and baking - results after 9, 12 and 15 months storage* (Report HEFH 80-3) (Unpublished data submitted to WHO by Wellcome Research Laboratories).

HANSEN, D.J., GOODMAN, L.R., MOORE, J.C., & HIGDON, P.K. (1983) Effects of the synthetic pyrethroids AC 222, 705, permethrin and fenvalerate on sheepshead minnows in early life stage of toxicity tests. *Environ. Toxicol. Chem.*, **2**: 251-258.

HART, D., BANHAM, P.B., GORE, C.W., PRATT, I., & WEIGHT, T.M. (1977c) *PP557: Liver hypertrophy study in rats-dietary administration over 26 weeks* (Report No. CTL/P/360) (Unpublished data submitted to WHO by ICI Central Toxicology Laboratory).

HELSON, B.V., KINGSBURY, P.D., & DE GROOT, P. (1986) The use of bioassays to assess aquatic arthropod mortality from permethrin drift deposits. *Aquat. Toxicol.*, **9**: 253-262.

HEND, R.W. & BUTTERWORTH, S.T.G. (1977) *Toxicity of insecticides: a short-term feeding study of WL 43379 in rats* (Report No. TLGR.0108.77) (Unpublished data submitted to WHO by Shell Research Ltd).

HENRIET, J., MARTIJN, A., & POLVISEN, H.H. (1985) *CIPAC Handbook. Volume 1C: Analysis of technical and formulated pesticides*, Hertfordshire, Collaborative International Pesticides Analytical Council Ltd, pp. 2172-2173.

HILL, E.F. & CAMARDESE, M.B. (1986) *Lethal dietary toxicities of environmental contaminants and pesticides to Coturnix*, Washington, DC, United States Department of the Interior, Fish and Wildlife Service, p.111 (Fish and Wildlife Technical Report No. 2).

HODGE, M.C.E., BANHAM, P.B., GLAISTER, J.R., RICHARDS, D., TAYLOR, K., & WEIGHT, T.M. (1977) *PP557: Three generation reproduction study in rats* (Unpublished report submitted to WHO by ICI Central Toxicology Laboratory).

HOGAN, G.K. & RINEHART, W.E. (1977) *A twenty-four month oral carcinogenicity study of FMC 33297 in mice* (Bio-Dynamics Inc. Project) (Unpublished report submitted to WHO by FMC Corporation).

HOLDWAY, D.A. & DIXON, D.G. (1988) Acute toxicity of permethrin or glyphosate pulse exposure to larval white sucker (*Catostomus commersoni*) and juvenile flagfish (*Jordanella floridae*) as modified by age and ration level. *Environ. Toxicol. Chem.*, **7**: 63-68.

HOLMSTEAD, R.L., CASIDA, J.E., RUZO, L.O., & FULLER, D.G. (1978) Pyrethroid photodecomposition: Permethrin. *J. agric. food Chem.*, **26**: 590-595.

HORIBA, M., KOBAYASHI, A., & MURANO, A. (1977) Gas-liquid chromatographic determination of a new pyrethroid, permethrin (S-3151) and its optical isomers. *Agric. biol. Chem.*, **41**: 581-586.

HOY, M.A., FLAHERTY, D., PEACOCK, W., & CULVER, D. (1979) Vineyard and laboratory evaluations of methomyl, dimethoate, and permethrin for a grape pest management program in the San Joaquin Valley of California. *J. econ. Entomol.*, **72**: 250-255.

HOYT, S.C., WESTIGARD, P.H., & BURTS, E.C. (1978) Effects of two synthetic pyrethroids on the codling moth, pear psylla, and various mite species in northwest apple and pear orchards. *J. econ. Entomol.*, **71**: 431-434.

HUNT, L.M. & GILBERT, B.N. (1977) Distribution and excretion rates of ^{14}C-labelled permethrin isomers administered orally to four lactating goats for 10 days. *J. agric. food Chem.*, **25**: 673-676.

HUNT, L.M., GILBERT, B.N., & LEMEILLEUR, C.A. (1979) Distribution and depletion of radioactivity in hens treated dermally with ^{14}C-labelled permethrin. *Poult. Sci.*, **58**: 1197-1201.

ISHMAEL, J. & LITCHFIELD, M.H. (1988) Chronic toxicity and carcinogenic evaluation of permethrin in rats and mice. *Fundam. appl. Toxicol.*, **11**: 308-311.

IVIE, G.W. & HUNT, L. (1980) Metabolites of *cis*- and *trans*-permethrin in lactating goats. *J. agric. food Chem.*, **28**: 1131-1138.

JAGGERS, S.E. & PARKINSON, G.R. (1979) *Permethrin: summary and review of acute toxicities in laboratory species* (Report No. CTL/P/461) (Unpublished data submitted to WHO by ICI Central Toxicology Laboratory).

JAMES, J.A. (1974) *Fetal toxicity study of 21Z73 (NRDC 143) in the rat* (Report No. BPAT 74-10) Bechenham, Wellcome Research Laboratories (Unpublished data submitted to WHO).

JAMES, J.A., (1979) *A multigeneration reproduction study of 21Z73 (permethrin) in the rat* (Report No. BPAT 79-3) Bechenham, Wellcome Research Laboratories (Unpublished data submitted to WHO).

JAMES, J.A., TAYLOR, P.E., & ROE, F.J.C. (1980) *Carcinogenicity study in mice with permethrin*, Bechenham, Wellcome Research Laboratories, (Report No. HEFG 80-29) (Unpublished data submitted to WHO).

JOLLY, A.L., Jr., AVAULT, J.W., Jr., KOONCE, K.L., & GRAVES, J.B. (1978) Acute toxicity of permethrin to several aquatic animals. *Trans. Am. Fish. Soc.*, **107**: 825-827.

JORDAN, E.G. & KAUFMAN, D.D. (1986) Degradation of *cis*- and *trans*-permethrin in flooded soil. *J. agric. food Chem.*, **34**: 880-884.

JORDAN, E.G., KAUFMAN, D.D., & KAYSER, A.J. (1982) The effect of soil temperature on the degradation of *cis*-, *trans*-permethrin in soil. *J. environ. Sci. Health*, **B 17**: 1-17.

KADOTA, T., MIYAMOTO, J., & ITO, N. (1975) *Six-month subacute oral toxicity of NRDC in Sprague-Dawley rats* (Unpublished data submitted to WHO by Sumitomo Chemical Co.).

KANEKO, H., OHKAWA, H., & MIYAMOTO, J. (1978) Degradation and movement of permethrin isomers in soil. *J. Pestic. Sci.*, **3**: 43-51.

KAUFMAN, D.D., HAYES, S.C., JORDAN, E.G., & KAYSER, A.J. (1977) Permethrin degradation in soil and microbial cultures. In: Elliott, M., ed. *Synthetic pyrethroids*, Washington, DC, American Chemical Society, pp. 147-161 (ACS symposium series 42).

KAUFMAN, D.D., RUSSEL, B.A., HELLING, C.S., & KAYSER, A.J. (1981) Movement of cypermethrin, deltamethrin, permethrin and their degradation products in soil. *J. agric. food Chem.*, **29**: 239-245.

KAUSHIK, N.K., STEPHENSON, G.L., SOLOMON, K.R., & DAY, K.E. (1985) Impact of permethrin on zooplankton communities in limnocorrals. *Can. J. Fish. aquat. Sci.*, **42**: 77-85.

KILLEEN, J.C. & RAPP, W.R. (1976a) *A three month oral toxicity study of FMC 33297 in Beagle dogs* (Bio-Dynamics Inc. Project) (Unpublished report submitted to WHO by FMC Corporation).

KILLEEN, J.C. & RAPP, W.R. (1976b) *A three month oral toxicity study of FMC 33297 in rats* (Bio-Dynamics Inc. Project) (Unpublished report submitted to WHO by FMC Corporation).

KINGSBURY, P.D. (1976) Effects of an aerial application of the synthetic pyrethroid permethrin on a forest stream. *Manitoba Entomol.*, **10**: 9-17.

KINGSBURY, P.D. & KREUTZWEISER, D.P. (1980a) *Environmental impact assessment of a semi-operational permethrin application*. Sault Ste. Marie, Ontario, Canada, Forest Pest Management Institute. Report No. FPM-X 30: pp.47.

KINGSBURY, P.D. & KREUTZWEISER, D.P. (1980b) *Dosage-effect studies on the impact of permethrin on trout streams*. Sault Ste. Marie, Ontario, Canada, Forest Pest Management Institute Report No. FPM-X 31.

KINGSBURY, P.D. & KREUTZWEISER, D.P. (1987) Permethrin treatments in Canadian forests. Part 1: Impact on fish. *Pestic. Sci.*, **19**: 35-48.

KOHDA, H., KADOTA, T., & MIYAMOTO, J. (1976a) *Teratogenic evaluation with permethrin in rats* (Unpublished report submitted to WHO by Sumitomo Chemical Co.).

KOHDA, H., KADOTA, T., & MIYAMOTO, J. (1976b) *Teratogenic evaluation with permethrin in mice* (Unpublished report submitted to WHO by Sumitomo Chemical Co.).

KOHDA, H., KADOTA, T., & MIYAMOTO, J. (1979a) *Acute oral, dermal and subcutaneous toxicities of permethrin in rats and mice* (Unpblished report submitted to WHO by Sumitomo Chemical Co.).

KOHDA, H., KANEDO, H., OHKAWA, H., KADOTA, T., & MIYAMOTO, J. (1979b) *Acute intraperitoneal toxicity of permethrin metabolites in mice* (Unpublished report submitted to WHO by Sumitomo Chemical Co.).

KOLMODIN-HEDMAN, B., SWENSSON, A., & AKERBLOM, M. (1982) Occupational exposure to some synthetic pyrethroids (permethrin and fenvalerate). *Arch. Toxicol.*, **50**: 27-33.

KREUTZWEISER, D.P. (1982) *The effects of permethrin on the invertebrate fauna of a Quebec forest.* Sault Ste Marie, Ontario, Canada, Forest Pest Management Institute, Report No. FPM-X 50: pp.44.

KREUTZWEISER, D.P. & KINGSBURY, P.D. (1987) Permethrin treatments in Canadian forests. Part 2: Impact on stream invertebrates. *Pestic. Sci.*, **19**: 49-60.

KUMARAGURU, A.K. & BEAMISH, F.W.H. (1981) Lethal toxicity of permethrin (NRDC-143) to rainbow trout, *Salmo gairdneri*, in relation to body weight and water temperature. *Water Res.*, **15**: 503-505.

KUMARAGURU, A.K., BEAMISH, F.W.H., & FERGUSON, H.W. (1982) Direct and circulatory paths of permethrin (NRDC-143) causing histopathological changes in the gills of rainbow trout, *Salmo gairdneri* Richardson. *J. Fish Biol.*, **20**: 87-91.

LAWRENCE, L.J. & CASIDA, J.E. (1982) Pyrethroid toxicology: Mouse intracerebral structure-toxicity relationship. *Pestic. Biochem. Physiol.*, **18**: 9-14.

LAWRENCE, L.J. & CASIDA, J.E. (1983) Stereospecific action of pyrethroid insecticides on the gamma-aminobutyric acid receptor-ionophore complex. *Science*, **221**: 1399-1401.

LAWRENCE, L.J., GEE, K.W., & YAMAMURA, H.I. (1985) Interactions of pyrethroid insecticides with chloride ionophore-associated binding sites. *Neurotoxicology*, **6**: 87-98.

LEAHEY, J.P. (1985) *The pyrethroid insecticides*, London, Taylor & Francis Ltd, p. 440.

LEAHEY, J.P. & CARPENTER, P.K. (1980) The uptake of metabolites of permethrin by plants grown in soil treated with [^{14}C]permethrin. *Pestic. Sci.*, **11**: 279-289.

LEAHEY, J.P., BEWICK, D.W., & SAUNDERS, R. (1977) *Accumulation and depletion of radioactive residues in the tissues of Mallard duck and Japanese quail following daily dosing with* ^{14}C-permethrin (Unpublished report submitted to WHO by ICI Plant Protection Division).

LE QUESNE, P.N., MAXWELL, I.C., & BUTTERWORTH, T.G. (1980) Transient facial sensory symptoms following exposure to synthetic pyrethroids: a clinical and electorophysiological assessment. *Neurotoxicology*, **2**: 1-11.

LINDEN, E., BENGTSSON, B.-E., SVANBERG, O., & SUNDSTROM, G. (1979) The acute toxicity of 78 chemicals and pesticide formulations against two brackish water organisms, the Bleak (*Alburnus alburnus*) and the *Nitocra spinipes*. *Chemosphere*, **11/12**: 843-851.

LINDQUIST, R.K., KRUEGER, H.R., & POWELL, C.C., Jr. (1987) Airborne and surface residues of permethrin after high- and low-volume applications in greenhouses. *J. environ. Sci. Health*, **B22**: 15-27.

LITCHFIELD, M.H. (1983) Characterisation of the principal mammalian toxicological and biological actions of synthetic pyrethroids. In: Miyamoto, J. & Kearney, P.C., ed. *Pesticide chemistry: human welfare and the environment. II. Natural products*, Oxford, Pergamon Press, pp. 207-211.

LONGSTAFF, E. (1976) *Permethrin: short-term predictive tests for carcinogenicity: results from the Ames test* (Report No. CTL/P/301) (Unpublished data submitted to WHO by ICI Central Toxicology Laboratory).

LORD, K.A., MCKINLEY, M., & WALKER, N. (1982) Degradation of permethrin in soils. *Environ. Pollut.* **A29**: 81-90.

LUND, A.E. & NARAHASHI, T. (1983) Kinetics of sodium channel modification as the basis for the variation in the nerve membrane effects of pyrethroids and DDT analogs. *Pestic. Biochem. Physiol.*, **20**: 203-216.

MCGREGOR, D.B. & WICKRAMARATNE, G.A., de S. (1976a) *Dominant lethal study in mice of ICI-PP557* (Report No. 623, Inveresk Research International Project No. 406722) (Unpublished data submitted to WHO by ICI Ltd).

MCGREGOR, D.B. & WICKRAMARATNE, G.A., de S. (1976b) *Teratogenicity study in rats of ICI-PP557* (Inveresk Research International Project No. 404898) (Unpublished data submitted to WHO by ICI Ltd.).

MCLEESE, D.W., METCALFE, C.D., & ZITKO, V. (1980) Lethality of permethrin, cypermethrin and fenvalerate to salmon, lobster and shrimp. *Bull. environ. Contam. Toxicol.*, **25**: 950-955.

MACPHEE, A., GAUL, S., & RAGAB, M.T.H. (1982) Control of blueberry thrips, *Frankliniella vaccinii* Morga, with permethrin and effect on yield and residue in fruit. *J. environ. Sci. Health*, **B17**: 183-193.

MCSHEEHY, T.W. & FINN, J.P. (1980) *21Z: Potential toxicity and oncogenicity in dietary administration to rats for a period of 104 weeks* (Report No. HEFG 80-33) (Unpublished data of Wellcome Research Laboratories).

MAREI, A.E.M., RUZO, L.O., & CASIDA, J.E. (1982) Analysis and persistence of permethrin, cypermethrin, deltamethrin and fenvalerate in the fat and brains of treated rats. *J. agric. food Chem.*, **30**: 558-562.

MATHUR, S.P., BELANGER, A., HAMILTON, H.A., & KHAN, S.U. (1980) Influence on microflora and persistence of field-applied disulfoton, permethrin and prometryne in an organic soil. *Pedobiologia*, **20**: 237-242.

MAYER, F.L., Jr. (1987) *Acute toxicity handbook of chemicals to estuarine organisms*, Springfield, Virginia, National Technical Information Service, p. 158 EPA/600/8-87/017.

MAYER, F.L., Jr. & ELLERSIECK, M.R. (1986) *Manual of acute toxicity: Interpretation and data base for 410 chemicals and 66 species of freshwater animals*, Washington, DC, United States Department of the Interior, Fish and Wildlife Service, pp.377-378.

MEISTER, R.T., BERG, G.L., SINE, C., MEISTER, S., & POPLYK, J. (1983) *Farm chemicals handbook. Section C. Pesticide dictionary*, Wilboughby, Ohio, Meister Publishing Co., pp. C180-C181.

METKER, L.W. (1978) *Subchronic inhalation toxicity of 3-(phenoxy-phenyl)methyl(+)-cis,trans-3-(2,2-dichloroethenyl)-2,2-dimethylcyclopropane-carboxylate (permethrin)*, Aberdeen Proving Ground, Maryland, US Army Environmental Hygiene Agency (Report No. 75-51-0026-80).

METKER, L.W., ANGERHOFER, R.A., POPE, C.R., & SWENTZEL, K.C. (1977) *Toxicology evaluation of 3-(phenoxyphenyl)methyl(+)-cis,trans-3-(2,2-dichloroethenyl)-2,2-dimethylcyclopropanecarboxylate (permethrin)*, Environmental Hygiene Agency (Report No. 75-51-0837-78).

MILLNER, C.K. & BUTTERWORTH, S.T.G. (1977) *Toxicity of pyrethroid insecticides: investigation of the neurotoxic potential of WL 43479 to adult hens*, (Report No. TLGR.0069.77) (Unpublished data submitted to WHO by Shell Research Ltd).

MIYAMOTO, J. (1976) Degradation, metabolism and toxicity of synthetic pyrethroids. *Environ. Health Perspect.*, **14**: 15-28.

MIYAMOTO, J. (1981) The chemistry, metabolism and residue analysis of synthetic pyrethroids, *Pure appl. Chem.*, **53**: 1967-2022.

MIYAMOTO, J. & KEARNEY, P.C. (1983) *Pesticide chemistry-human welfare and the environment. Proceedings of the Fifth International Congress of Pesticide Chemistry, Kyoto, Japan, 29 August-4 September 1982*, Oxford, Pergamon Press, Vol. 1-4.

MULLA, M.S., DARWAZEH, H.A., & MAJORI, G. (1975) Field efficacy of some promising mosquito larvicides and their effect on nontarget organisms. *Mosq. News,* **35**: 179-185.

MULLA, M.S., NAVVAB-GOJRATI, H.A., & DARWAZEH, H.A. (1978a) Toxicity of mosquito larvicidal pyrethroids to four species of freshwater fishes. *Environ. Entomol.,* **7**: 428-430.

MULLA, M.S., NAVVAB-GOJRATI, H.A., & DARWAZEH, H.A. (1978b) Biological activity and longevity of new synthetic pyrethroids against mosquitoes and some nontarget insects. *Mosq. News,* **38**: 90-96.

MULLA, M.S., DARWAZEH, H.A., & DHILLON, K.S. (1981) Impact and joint action of decamethrin and permethrin and freshwater fishes on mosquitoes. *Bull. environ. Contam. Toxicol.,* **26**: 689-695.

NASSIF, M., BROOKE, J.P., HUTCHINSON, D.B.A., & KAMEL, O.M. (1980) Studies with permethrin against body lice in Egypt. *Pestic. Sci.,* **11**: 679-684.

NEWELL, G.W. & SKINNER W.A. (1976) *In vitro microbiological mutagenicity study of an FMC corporation compound* (Unpublished report submitted to WHO by FMC Corporation).

NOMURA, Y. & SEGAWA, T. (1979) *Pharmacological study of permethrin: effects of isolated ileum, nictitating membrane, respiration, blood pressure and electrocardiography* (Unpublished report submitted to WHO by Sumitomo Chemical Co.).

OHKAWA, H., KANEKO, H., & MIYAMOTO, J. (1977) Metabolism of permethrin in bean plants. *J. Pestic. Sci.,* **2**: 67-76.

OHSHIMA, M., TAKIMOTO, Y., & MATSUDA, T. (1988) *Accumulation and metabolism of ^{14}C-permethrin in carp (Cyprinus carpio)* (Unpublished data submitted to WHO by Sumitomo Chemical Co.).

OKUNO, Y., MIYAGAWA, H., HOSOI, R., & KADOTA, T. (1976) *Skin and eye irritation study of permethrin (S-3151) in rabbits* (Unpublished report submitted to WHO by Sumitomo Chemical Co.).

PARKINSON, G.R. (1978) *Permethrin: acute toxicity to male rats* (Report No. CTL/P/388) (Unpublished data submitted to WHO by ICI Central Toxicology Laboratory).

PARKINSON, G.R., BERRY, P.N., GLAISTER, J., GORE, C.W., LEFEVRE, V.K., & MURPHY, J.A. (1976) *PP557 (Permethrin): acute and sub-acute toxicity,* (Report No. CTL/P/225) (Unpublished data submitted to WHO by ICI Central Toxicology Laboratory).

PAYNTER, O.C., BUDD, E.R., & LITT, B.D. (1982) *Permethrin. Assessment of chronic and oncogenic effects: A summary*, Washington, DC, Toxicology Branch, Hazard Evaluation Division, Office of Pesticide Programs, US Environmental Protection Agency (Unpublished data submitted to WHO).

PEGUM, J.S. & DOUGHTY, B.J. (1978) *Human skin patch test with pyrethrins, kadethrin, permethrin and decamethrin*, Berkhamsted Hill, Wellcome Group Research and Development (Report No. NEFJ 78-2) (Unpublished data submitted to WHO).

PIERCY, D.W.T., REYNOLDS, J., & JAMES, J.A. (1976) *Effects of diet on the acute toxicity of permethrin in the female rat*, Berkhamsted Hill, Wellcome Research and Development (Report no. 77-11) (Unpublished data submitted to WHO).

PIKE, K.S., MAYER, D.F., GLAZER, M., & KIOUS, C. (1982) Effects of permethrin on mortality and foraging behavior of honey bees in sweet corn. *Environ. Entomol.*, **11**: 951-953.

PLAPP, F.W., Jr & BULL, D.L. (1978) Toxicity and selectivity of some insecticides to *Chrysopa carnea*, a predator of the tobacco budworm. *Environ. Entomol.*, **7**: 431-434.

PLAPP, F.W., Jr & VINSON, S.B. (1977) Comparative toxicities of some insecticides to the tobacco budworm and its ichneumonid parasite, *Campoletis sonorensis*. *Environ. Entomol.*, **6**: 381-384.

PLUIJMEN, M., DREVON, C., MONTESANO, R., MALAVEILLE, C., HAUTEFEUILLE, A., & BARTSCH, H. (1984) Lack of mutagenicity of synthetic pyrethroids in Salmonella typhimurium strains in V79 Chinese hamster cells. *Mutat. Res.*, **137**: 7-15.

RACEY, P.A. & SWIFT, S.M. (1986) The residual effect of remedial timber treatments on bats. *Biol. Conserv.*, **35**: 205-214.

RAPP, W.R. (1978) *Twenty-four month oral toxicity/oncogenicity study of FMC33297 in mice. Histopathology report* (Unpublished data of FMC Corporation).

REYNOLDS, J., PIERCY, D.W.T., CLAMPITT, R.B., JAMES, J.A., THOMPSON, P.M., FAREBROTHER, D.A., & DAYAN, A.D. (1978) *Permethrin oral administration to dogs for 6 months*, Berkhamsted Hill, Wellcome Research Laboratories (Report No. HEFG 78-14) (Unpublished data submitted to WHO).

RICHARDS, D., BANHAM, P.B., KILMARTIN, M., & WEIGHT, T.M. (1980) *Permethrin: Teratogenicity study in the rabbit* (Report No. CTL/P/523) (Unpublished report submitted to WHO by ICI Ltd).

RISHIKESH, N., CLARKE, J.L., MATHIN, H.L., KING, J.S., & PEARSON, J. (1978) *Evaluation of decamethrins and permethrin against Anopheles gambiae and Anopheles funestus in a village trial in Nigeria* (WHO/VBC/78.679) (Unpublished report of Division of Vector Biology Control, World Health Organization).

ROBERTS, T.R. & WRIGHT, A.N. (1981) The metabolism of 3-phenoxybenzyl alcohol, a pyrethroid metabolite, in plants. *Pestic. Sci.*, 12: 161-169.

ROCK, G.C. (1979) Relative toxicity of two synthetic pyrethroids to a predator *Amblyseius fallacis* and its prey *Tetranychus urticae*. *J. econ. Entomol.*, 72: 293-294.

ROSS, D.B. & PRENTICE, D.E. (1977) *Examination of permethrin (PP557) for neurotoxicity in the domestic hen*, Huntingdon, Huntingdon Research Centre (Report No. ICI/157-NT/77468) (Unpublished data submitted to WHO by FMC Corporation and ICI Ltd).

ROSS, D.B., CAMERON, D.M., & ROBERTS, N.L. (1976a) *The acute oral toxicity (LD_{50}) of PP557 (permethrin) to Mallard ducks*, Huntingdon, Huntingdon Research Centre (Report No. ICI 68/WL/7639) (Unpublished data submitted to WHO by ICI Ltd).

ROSS, D.B., CAMERON, D.M., & ROBERTS, N.L. (1976b) *The sub-acute toxicty (LC_{50}) of PP557 (permethrin) to Mallard ducks*, Huntingdon, Huntingdon Research Centre (Report No. ICI 68/WL/75837) (Unpublished data submitted to WHO by ICI Ltd).

ROSS, D.B., CAMERON, D.M., & ROBERTS, N.L. (1976c) *The acute oral toxicity (LD_{50}) of PP557 (permethrin) to Starling*, Huntingdon, Huntingdon Research Centre (Report No. ICI 68/WL/7637) (Unpublished data submitted to WHO by ICI Ltd).

ROSS, D.B., CAMERON, D.M., & ROBERTS, N.L. (1976d) *The sub-acute toxicity (LC_{50}) of PP557 (permethrin) to Starling*, Huntingdon, Huntingdon Research Centre (Report No. ICI 68/WL/7636) (Unpublished data submitted to WHO by ICI Ltd).

ROSS, D.B., CAMERON, D.M., & ROBERTS, N.L. (1976e) *The sub-acute toxicity (LC_{50}) of PP557 (permethrin) to Ring-necked pheasant*, Huntingdon, Huntingdon Research Centre (Report No. ICI 68/WL/75839) (Unpublished data submitted to WHO by ICI Ltd).

ROSS, D.B., CAMERON, D.M., & ROBERTS, N.L. (1977a) *The acute oral toxicity (LD_{50}) of PP557 (permethrin) to Ring-necked pheasant*, Huntingdon, Huntingdon Research Centre (Report No. ICI 68/WL/77154) (Unpublished data submitted to WHO by ICI Ltd).

ROSS, D.B., PRENTICE, D.E., MAJEED, S.K., GIBSON, W.A., CAMERON, D.M., CAMERON, M. McD., & ROBERTS, N.L. (1977b) *The incorporation of permethrin in the diet of laying hens (part I)*, Huntingdon, Huntingdon Research Centre (Report No. ICI 152/77387) (Unpublished data submitted to WHO by ICI Ltd).

ROUSH, R.T. & HOY, M.A. (1978) Relative toxicity of permethrin to a predator, *Metaseiulus occidentalis*, and its prey, *Tetranychus urticae*. *Environ. Entomol.*, **7**: 287-288.

RUIGT, G.S.F. & VAN DEN BERCKEN, J. (1986) Action of pyrethroids on a nerve-muscle preparation of the clawed frog, *Xenopus laevis*. *Pestic. Biochem. Physiol.*, **25**: 176-187.

SASINOVICH, L.M. & PANSHINA, T.N. (1987) [Substantiation of hygienic rules for synthetic pyrethroid content in the work zone air]. *Gig. Tr. prof. Zabol.*, **8**: 48-50 (in Russian).

SCHROEDER, R.E. & RINEHART, W.E. (1977) *A three generation reproduction study of FMC33297 in rats* (Bio-Dynamics Inc Project) (Unpublished report submitted to WHO by FMC Corporation).

SHAH, P.V., MONROE, R.J., & GUTHRIE, F.E. (1981) Comparative rates of dermal penetration of insecticides in mice. *Toxicol. appl. Pharmacol.*, **59**: 414-423.

SHAROM, M.S. & SOLOMON, K.R. (1981) Adsorption-desorption, degradation, and distribution of permethrin in aqueous systems. *J. agric. food Chem.*, **29**: 1122-1125.

SHERMAN, R.A. (1979) *Preliminary behavioural assessment of habituation to the insecticide permethrin*, Aberdeen Proving Ground, Maryland, US Army Environmental Hygiene Agency (Report No. 75-51-002679).

SHIRASU, Y., MORIYA, M., & OTA, T. (1979) *Mutagenicity of S-3151 in bacterial test systems* (Unpublished report submitted to WHO by Sumitomo Chemical Co.).

SHONO, T., OHSAWA, K., & CASIDA, J.E. (1979) Metabolism of *trans*- and *cis*-permethrin, *trans*- and *cis*-cypermethrin, and decamethrin by microsomal enzymes. *J. agric. food Chem.*, **27**: 316-325.

SHOUR, M.H. & CROWDER, L.A. (1980) Effects of pyrethroid insecticides on the common green lacewing. *J. econ. Entomol.*, **73**: 306-309.

SIEGEL, M.M., HILDEBRAND, B.E., & HALL, D.R. (1980) Determination of permethrin in environmental waters by gas chromatography-selected ion monitoring-mass spectroscopy using ion counting detection. *Int. J. environ. anal. Chem.*, **8**: 107-126.

SIMMON, V.F. (1976) *In vitro microbiological mutagenicity study of an FMC corporation compound,* Menlo Park, Stanford Research Institute, (Report No. LSC-4768) (Unpublished report submitted to WHO).

SIMONAITIS, R.A. & CAIL, R.S. (1977) Gas chromatographic determination of residues of the synthetic pyrethroid FMC33297. In: Elliott, M., ed. *Synthetic pyrethroids,* Washington, DC, American Chemical Society, pp. 211-223 (ACS Symposium Series U2).

SODERLUND, D.M. & CASIDA, J.E. (1977) Effects of pyrethroid structure on rate of hydrolysis and oxidation by mouse liver microsomal enzymes. *Pestic. Biochem. Physiol.,* 7: 391-401.

SPENCER, F. & BERHANCE, Z. (1982) Uterine and fetal characteristics in rats following a post-implantational exposure to permethrin. *Bull. environ. Contam. Toxicol.,* 29: 84-88.

STAATZ, C.G., BLOOM, A.S., & LECH, J.J. (1982) A pharmacological study of pyrethroid neurotoxicity in mice. *Pestic. Biochem. Physiol.,* **17**: 287-292.

STEVENSON, J.H., NEEDHAM, P.H., & WALKER, J. (1978) *Poisoning of honeybee by pesticides: Investigation of the changing pattern in Britain over 20 years.* Rothamsted Experimental Station Report (1977), Part 2: 55-72.

STRATTON, G.W. & CORKE, C.T. (1981) Interaction of permethrin with *Daphnia magna* in the presence and absence of particulate material. *Environ. Pollut.,* **A24**: 135-144.

STRATTON, G.W. & CORKE, C.T. (1982) Toxicity of the insecticide permethrin and some degradation products towards algae and cyanobacteria. *Environ. Pollut.* **A29**: 71-80.

SUNDARAM, K.M.S., DE GROOT, P., & SUNDARAM, A. (1987) Permethrin deposits and airborne concentrations downwind from a single swath application using a back pack mist blower. *J. environ. Sci. Health,* **B22**: 171-193.

SUZUKI, H. (1977) *Studies on the mutagenicity of some pyrethroids on salmonella strains in the presence of mouse hepatic S9 fractions* (Unpublished report submitted to WHO by Sumitomo Chemical Co.).

SWAINE, H. & SAPIETS, A. (1981a) *Cypermethrin: residue transfer study with dairy cows fed on a diet containing the insecticide* (Report No. RJ0186B) (Unpublished data submitted to WHO by ICI Ltd).

SWAINE, H. & SAPIETS, A. (1981b) *Cypermethrin: residue levels of the major metabolites of the insecticide in the milk and tissues of dairy cows fed on a diet containing cypermethrin at 50 mg/kg* (Report No. RJ0198B) (Unpublished data submitted to WHO by ICI Ltd).

SWAINE, H., EDWARD, M.J., & USSARY, J.P. (1978) *Permethrin crop protection study* (Report No. TMV 0378B) (Unpublished data submitted to WHO by ICI Ltd).

TAKAHASHI, K., OKUDA, No., & SHIRASU, Y. (1979) *Effects of permethrin on hexobarbital induced sleeping time in mice and electró-encephalography in rabbits* (Unpublished report submitted to WHO by Sumitomo Chemical Co.).

TYLER, J.F.C. (1987) Gas chromatographic method for determination of permethrin in pesticide formulations: Collaborative study. *J. Assoc. Off. Anal. Chem.*, **70**(1): 53-55.

US EPA (1981) *Advisary opinion on the oncogenic potential of permethrin*, Washington, DC, US Environmental Protection Agency (Unpublished report submitted to WHO).

USSARY, J.P. (1979) *Permethrin residues on sweet corn* (Report No. TMU0438B) (Unpublished data submitted to WHO by ICI Americas Inc.).

USSARY, J.P. (1978) *Permethrin residues on sweet corn* (Report No. TMU0413B) (Unpublished data submitted to WHO by ICI Americas Inc.).

USSARY, J.P. & BRAITHWAITE, G.B. (1980) *Residues of permethrin and 3-phenoxy-benzyl alcohol in cow tissues* (Trial No. 35NC79-001. Report No. TMU0493B) (Unpublished data submitted to WHO by ICI Americas Inc.).

VAN DEN BERCKEN, J. (1977) The action of allethrin on the peripheral nervous system of the frog. *Pestic. Sci.*, **8**: 692-699.

VAN DEN BERCKEN, J. & VIJVERBERG, H.P.M. (1980a) Voltage clamp studies on the effects of allethrin and DDT on the sodium channels in frog myelinated nerve membrane. In: *Insect neurobiology and pesticide action*, London, Society of Chemical Industry, pp. 79-85.

VAN DEN BERCKEN, J. & VIJVERBERG, H.P.M. (1980b) Effects of insecticides on the sensory system of Xenopus. In: *Insect neurobiology and pesticide action*, London, Society of Chemical Industry, pp.391-397.

VAN DEN BERCKEN, J., AKKERMANS, L.M.A., & VAN DER ZALM, J.M., (1973) DDT-like action of allethrin in the sensory nervous system of *Xenopus laevis*. *Eur. J. Pharmacol.*, **21**: 95-106.

VAN DEN BERCKEN, J., KROESE, A.B.A., & AKKERMANS, L.M.A. (1979) Effect of insecticides on the sensory nervous system. In: Narahashi, T., ed. *Neurotoxicology of insecticides and pheromones*, New York, London, Plenum Press, pp. 183-210.

VERSCHOYLE, R.D. & ALDRIDGE, W.N. (1980) Structure-activity relationship of some pyrethrins to rats. *Arch. Toxicol.*, **45**: 325-329.

VIJVERBERG, H.P.M. & VAN DEN BERCKEN, J. (1979) Frequency-dependent effects of the pyrethroid insecticide decamethrin in frog myelinated nerve fibres. *Eur. J. Phamacol.*, **58**: 501-504.

VIJVERBERG, H.P.M. & VAN DEN BERCKEN, J. (1982) Action of pyrethroid insecticides on the vertebrate nervous system. *Neuropathol. appl. Neurobiol.*, **8**: 421-440.

VIJVERBERG, H.P.M., RUIGT, G.S.F., & VAN DEN BERCKEN, J. (1982a) Structure-related effects of pyrethroid insecticides on the lateral-line sense organ and on peripheral nerves of the clawed frog, *Xenopus laevis*. *Pestic. Biochem. Physiol.*, **18**: 315-324.

VIJVERBERG, H.P.M., VAN DER ZALM, J.M., & VAN DEN BERCKEN, J. (1982b) Similar mode of action of pyrethroids and DDT on sodium channel gating in mylinated nerves. *Nature (Lond.)*, **295**: 601-603.

VIJVERBERG, H.P.M., VAN DER ZALM, J.M., VAN KLEEF, R.G.D.M., & VAN DEN BERCKEN, J. (1983) Temperature and structure-dependent interaction of pyrethroids with the sodium channels in frog node of Ranvier. *Biochim. Biophys. Acta*, **728**: 73-82.

WALLWORK, L.M. & MALONE, J.C. (1974) *21Z73 (25:75) effect of different solvents on the rat oral toxicity* (Report No. HEFG 75-4) Berkhamsted, Wellcome Research Laboratories (Unpublished data submitted to WHO).

WALLWORK, L.M., CLAMPITT, R.B., & MALONE, J.C. (1974a) *10-day cumulative oral toxicity study with 21Z73 in mice*, Berkhamsted, Wellcome Research Laboratories (Report No. HEFG 74-9) (Unpublished data submitted to WHO).

WALLWORK, L.M., CLAMPITT, R.B., & MALONE, J.C. (1974b) *10-day cumulative oral toxicity study with 21Z73 in rats*, Berkhamsted, Wellcome Research Laboratories (Unpublished report submitted to WHO).

WELLS, D., GRAYSON, B.T., & LANGNER, E. (1986) Vapour pressure of permethrin. *Pestic. Sci.*, **17**: 473-476.

WHO (1979) WHO Technical Report Series, No. 634 (Safe use of pesticides. Third Report of the WHO Expert Committee on Vector Biology and Control), pp. 18-23.

WHO (1988) *The WHO recommended classification of pesticides by hazard: Guidelines to classification 1988-89*, Geneva, World Health Organization (Unpublished report VBC/88.953).

WHO/FAO (1984) *Data sheet on pesticides No. 51: Permethrin,* Geneva, World Health Organization (VBC/DS/84.51).

WILLIAMS, I.H. & BROWN, M.J. (1979) Persistence of permethrin and WL 43775 in soil. *J. agric. food Chem.,* **27**: 130-132.

WOODRUFF, R.C., PHILLIPS, J.P., & IRWIN, D. (1983) Pesticide-induced complete and partial chromosome loss in screens with repair-defective females of *Drosophila melanogaster. Environ. Mutagen.,* **5**: 835-846.

WOOD, MACKENZIE & Co. (1980) Pyrethroids. *Agrochem. Monit.,* **9**: 3-14.

WOOD, MACKENZIE & Co. (1981) Pyrethroids. *Agrochem. Monit.,* **15**: 3-27.

WOOD, MACKENZIE & Co. (1982) Pyrethroids. *Agrochem. Monit.,* **21**: 3-17.

WOOD, MACKENZIE & Co. (1983) Pyrethroids. *Agrochem. Monit.,* **27**: 3-12.

WOOD, MACKENZIE & Co. (1984) Pyrethroids. *Agrochem. Monit.,* **33**: 2-12.

WORKMAN, R.B. (1977) Pesticides toxic to striped earwig, an important insect predator. *Proc. Florida State Hortic. Soc.,* **90**: 401-402.

WORTHING, C.R. & WALKER, S.B. (1983) *The pesticide manual,* 7th ed., Croydon, British Crop Protection Council, p. 427.

WORTHING, C.R. & WALKER, S.B. (1987) Permethrin. In: *The pesticide manual,* 8th ed., Croydon, British Crop Protection Council, pp. 647-648.

WOUTERS, W. & VAN DEN BERCKEN, J. (1978) Action of pyrethroids. *Gen. Pharmacol.,* **9**: 387-398.

ZITKO, V., CARSON, W.G., & METCALFE, C.D. (1977) Toxicity of pyrethroids to juvenile atlantic salmon. *Bull. environ. Contam. Toxicol.,* **18**: 35-41.

ZITKO, V., MCLEESE, D.W., METCALFE, C.D., & CARSON, W.G. (1979) Toxicity of permethrin, decamethrin, and related pyrethroids to salmon and lobster. *Bull. environ. Contam. Toxicol.,* **21**: 338-343.

APPENDIX I

On the basis of electrophysiological studies with peripheral nerve preparations of frogs (*Xenopus laevis; Rana temporaria*, and *Rana esculenta*), it is possible to distinguish between 2 classes of pyrethroid insecticides: (Type I and Type II). A similar distinction between these 2 classes of pyrethroids has been made on the basis of the symptoms of toxicity in mammals and insects (Van den Bercken et al., 1979; WHO, 1979; Verschoyle & Aldridge, 1980; Glickman & Casida, 1982; Lawrence & Casida, 1982). The same distinction was found in studies on cockroaches (Gammon et al., 1981).

Based on the binding assay on the gamma-aminobutyric acid (GABA) receptor-ionophore complex, synthetic pyrethroids can also be classified into two types: the α-cyano-3-phenoxybenzyl pyrethroids and the non-cyano pyrethroids (Gammon et al., 1982; Gammon & Casida, 1983; Lawrence & Casida, 1983; Lawrence et al., 1985).

Pyrethroids that do not contain an α-cyano group (allethrin, d-phenothrin, permethrin, tetramethrin, cismethrin, and bioresmethrin) (Type I: T-syndrome)

The pyrethroids that do not contain an α-cyano group give rise to pronounced repetitive activity in sense organs and in sensory nerve fibres (Van den Bercken et al., 1973). At room temperature, this repetitive activity usually consists of trains of 3-10 impulses and occasionally up to 25 impulses. Train duration is between 10 and 5 milliseconds.

These compounds also induce pronounced repetitive firing of the presynaptic motor nerve terminal in the neuromuscular junction (Van den Bercken, 1977). There was no significant effect of the insecticide on neurotransmitter release or on the sensitivity of the subsynaptic membrane, nor on the muscle fibre membrane. Presynaptic repetitive firing was also observed in the sympathetic ganglion treated with these pyrethroids.

In the lateral-line sense organ and in the motor nerve terminal, but not in the cutaneous touch receptor or in sensory nerve fibres, the pyrethroid-induced repetitive activity increases dramatically as the temperature is lowered, and a decrease of 5°C in temperature may cause a more than 3-fold increase in the number of repetitive impulses per train. This effect is easily reversed by raising the temperature. The origin of this "negative temperature coefficient" is not clear (Vijverberg et al., 1983).

Synthetic pyrethroids act directly on the axon through interference with the sodium channel gating mechanism that underlies the generation and conduction of each nerve impulse. The transitional state of the sodium channel is controlled by 2 separately acting gating mechanisms, referred to as the activation gate and the inactivation gate. Since pyrethroids only appear to affect the sodium current during depolarization, the rapid opening of the activation gate and the slow closing of the inactivation gate proceed normally. However, once the sodium channel is open, the activation gate is restrained in the open position by the pyrethroid molecule. While all pyrethroids have essentially the same basic mechanism of action, however, the rate of relaxation differs substantially for the various pyrethroids (Flannigan & Tucker, 1985).

In the isolated node of Ranvier, allethrin causes prolongation of the transient increase in sodium permeability of the nerve membrane during excitation (Van den Bercken & Vijverberg, 1980a,b). Evidence so far available indicates that allethrin selectively slows down the closing of the activation gate of a fraction of the sodium channels that open during depolarization of the membrane. The time constant of closing of the activation gate in the allethrin-affected channels is about 100 milliseconds compared with less than 100 microseconds in the normal sodium channel, i.e. it is slowed down by a factor of more than 100. This results in a marked prolongation of the sodium current across the nerve membrane during excitation, and this prolonged sodium current is directly responsible for the repetitive activity induced by allethrin (Vijverberg et al., 1983).

The effects of cismethrin on synaptic transmission in the frog neuromuscular junction, as reported by Evans (1976), are almost identical to those of allethrin, i.e. presynaptic repetitive firing, and no significant effects on transmitter release or on the subsynaptic membrane.

Interestingly, the action of these pyrethroids closely resembles that of the insecticide DDT in the peripheral nervous system of the frog. DDT also causes pronounced repetitive activity in sense organs, in sensory nerve fibres, and in motor nerve terminals, due to a prolongation of the transient increase in sodium permeability of the nerve membrane during excitation. Recently, it was demonstrated that allethrin and DDT have essentially the same effect on sodium channels in frog myelinated nerve membrane. Both compounds slow down the rate of closing of a fraction of the sodium channels that open on depolarization of the membrane (Van den Bercken et al., 1973, 1979; Vijverberg et al., 1982b).

In the electrophysiological experiments using giant axons of crayfish, the type I pyrethroids and DDT analogues retain sodium channels in a modified open state only intermittently, cause large depolarizing after-potentials, and evoke repetitive firing with minimal effect on the resting potential (Lund & Narahashi, 1983).

These results strongly suggest that permethrin and cismethrin, like allethrin, primarily affect the sodium channels in the nerve membrane and cause a prolongation of the transient increase in sodium permeability of the membrane during excitation.

The effects of pyrethroids on end-plate and muscle action potentials were studied in the pectoralis nerve-muscle preparation of the clawed frog (*Xenopus laevis*). Type I pyrethroids (allethrin, cismethrin, bioresmethrin, and 1R,*cis*-phenothrin) caused moderate presynaptic repetitive activity, resulting in the occurrence of multiple end-plate potentials (Ruigt & Van den Bercken, 1986).

Pyrethroids with an α-cyano group on the 3-phenoxybenzyl alcohol (deltamethrin, cypermethrin, cyhalothrin, lambda-cyhalothrin, fenvalerate, and fenpropanate) (Type II: CS-syndrome)

The pyrethroids with an α-cyano group cause an intense repetitive activity in the lateral line organ in the form of long-lasting trains of impulses (Vijverberg et al., 1982a). Such a train may last for up to 1 min and contains thousands of impulses. The duration of the trains and the number of impulses per train increase markedly on lowering the temperature. Cypermethrin does not cause repetitive activity in myelinated nerve fibres. Instead, this pyrethroid causes a frequency-dependent depression of the nervous impulse, brought about by a progressive depolarization of the nerve membrane as a result of the summation of depolarizing after-potentials during train stimulation (Vijverberg & Van den Bercken, 1979; Vijverberg et al., 1983).

In the isolated node of Ranvier, cypermethrin, like allethrin, specifically affects the sodium channels of the nerve membrane and causes a long-lasting prolongation of the transient increase in sodium permeability during excitation, presumably by slowing down the closing of the activation gate of the sodium channel (Vijverberg & Van den Bercken, 1979; Vijverberg et al., 1983). The time constant of closing of the activation gate in the cypermethrin-affected channels is prolonged to more than 100 milliseconds. Apparently, the amplitude of the prolonged sodium current after cypermethrin is too small to induce repetitive activity in nerve fibres, but is sufficient to cause the long-lasting repetitive firing in the lateral-line sense organ.

These results suggest that α-cyano pyrethroids primarily affect the sodium channels in the nerve membrane and cause a long-lasting prolongation of the transient increase in sodium permeability of the membrane during excitation.

In the electrophysiological experiments using giant axons of crayfish, the Type II pyrethroids retain sodium channels in a modified continuous open state persistently, depolarize the membrane, and block the action potential without causing repetitive firing (Lund & Narahashi, 1983).

Diazepam, which facilitates GABA reaction, delayed the onset of action of deltamethrin and fenvalerate, but not permethrin and allethrin, in both the mouse and cockroach. Possible mechanisms of the Type II pyrethroid syndrome include action at the GABA receptor complex or a closely linked class of neuroreceptor (Gammon et al., 1982).

The Type II syndrome of intracerebrally administered pyrethroids closely approximates that of the convulsant picrotoxin (PTX). Deltamethrin inhibits the binding of [^{3}H]-dihydropicrotoxin to rat brain synaptic membranes, whereas the non-toxic R epimer of deltamethrin is inactive. These findings suggest a possible relation between the Type II pyrethroid action and the GABA receptor complex. The stereospecific correlation between the toxicity of Type II pyrethroids and their potency to inhibit the [^{35}S]-TBPS binding was established using a radioligand, [^{35}S]-*t*-butyl-bicyclophosphorothionate [^{35}S]-TBPS. Studies with 37 pyrethroids revealed an absolute correlation, without any false positive or negative, between mouse intracerebral toxicity and *in vitro* inhibition: all toxic cyano compounds including deltamethrin, 1R,*cis*-cypermethrin, 1R,*trans*-cypermethrin, and [2S,αS]-fenvalerate were inhibitors, but their non-toxic stereoisomers were not; non-cyano pyrethroids were much less potent or were inactive (Lawrence & Casida, 1983).

In the [^{35}S]-TBPS and [^{3}H]-Ro 5-4864 (a convulsant benzodiazepine radioligand) binding assay, the inhibitory potencies of pyrethroids were closely related to their mammalian toxicities. The most toxic pyrethroids of Type II were the most potent inhibitors of [^{3}H]-Ro 5-4864 specific binding to rat brain membranes. The [^{3}H]-dihydropicrotoxin and [^{35}S]-TBPS binding studies with pyrethroids strongly indicated that Type II effects of pyrethroids are mediated, at least in part, through an interaction with a GABA-regulated chloride ionophore-associated binding site. Moreover, studies with [^{3}H]-Ro 5-4864 support this hypothesis and, in addition, indicate that the pyrethroid-binding site may be very closely related to the convulsant benzodiazepine site of action (Lawrence et al., 1985).

The Type II pyrethroids (deltamethrin, 1R, *cis*-cypermethrin and [2S,αS]-fenvalerate) increased the input resistance of crayfish claw opener muscle fibres bathed in GABA. In contrast, two non-insecticidal stereoisomers and Type I pyrethroids (permethrin, resmethrin, allethrin) were inactive. Therefore, cyanophenoxybenzyl pyrethroids appear to act on the GABA receptor-ionophore complex (Gammon & Casida, 1983).

The effects of pyrethroids on end-plate and muscle action potentials were studied in the pectoralis nerve-muscle preparation of the clawed frog (*Xenopus laevis*). Type II pyrethroids (cypermethrin and deltamethrin) induced trains of repetitive muscle action potentials without presynaptic repetitive activity. However, an intermediate group of pyrethroids (1R-permethrin, cyphenothrin, and fenvalerate) caused both types of effect. Thus, in muscle or nerve membrane the pyrethroid induced repetitive activities due to a prolongation of the sodium current. But no clear distinction was observed between non-cyano and α-cyano pyrethroids (Ruigt & Van den Bercken, 1986).

Appraisal

In summary, the results strongly suggest that the primary target site of pyrethroid insecticides in the vertebrate nervous system is the sodium channel in the nerve membrane. Pyrethroids without an α-cyano group (allethrin, d-phenothrin, permethrin, and cismethrin) cause a moderate prolongation of the transient increase in sodium permeability of the nerve membrane during excitation. This results in relatively short trains of repetitive nerve impulses in sense organs, sensory (afferent) nerve fibres, and, in effect, nerve terminals. On the other hand, the α-cyano pyrethroids cause a long-lasting prolongation of the transient increase in sodium permeability of the nerve membrane during excitation. This results in long-lasting trains of repetitive impulses in sense organs and a frequency-dependent depression of the nerve impulse in nerve fibres. The difference in effects between permethrin and cypermethrin, which have identical molecular structures except for the presence of an α-cyano group on the phenoxybenzyl alcohol, indicates that it is this α-cyano group that is responsible for the long-lasting prolongation of the sodium permeability.

Since the mechanisms responsible for nerve impulse generation and conduction are basically the same throughout the entire nervous system, pyrethroids may also induce repetitive activity in various parts of the brain. The difference in symptoms of poisoning by α-cyano pyrethroids, compared with the classical pyrethroids, is not necessarily due to an exclusive central site of action. It may be related to the long-lasting repetitive activity in sense organs and possibly in other parts of the nervous system, which, in a more advance state of poisoning, may be accompanied by a frequency-dependent depression of the nervous impulse.

Pyrethroids also cause pronounced repetitive activity and a prolongation of the transient increase in sodium permeability of the nerve membrane in insects and other invertebrates. Available information indicates that the sodium channel in the nerve membrane is also the most important target site of pyrethroids in the invertebrate nervous system (Wouters & Van den Bercken, 1978; WHO, 1979).

Because of the universal character of the processes underlying nerve excitability, the action of pyrethroids should not be considered restricted to particular animal species, or to a certain region of the nervous system. Although it has been established that sense organs and nerve endings are the most vulnerable to the action of pyrethroids, the ultimate lesion that causes death will depend on the animal species, environmental conditions, and on the chemical structure and physical characteristics of the pyrethroid molecule (Vijverberg & Van den Bercken, 1982).

RESUME, EVALUATION, CONLUSIONS ET RECOMMANDATIONS

1. Résumé et Evaluation

1.1 Identité, propriétés physicochimiques et méthodes d'analyse

La perméthrine, un pyréthroide photostable, a été synthétisée pour la première fois en 1973 et commercialisée en 1977. C'est un ester de l'analogue dichloré de l'acide chrysanthémique, à savoir l'acide (dichloro-2,2 vinyl)-3 diméthyl-2,2 cyclopropanecarboxylique (Cl_2CA) et de l'alcool phénoxy-3 benzylique. Les produits techniques se présentent sous la forme d'un mélange de quatre stéréoisomères ayant les configurations [1R,trans], [1R,cis], [1S,trans] et [1S,cis] dans les proportions approximatives de 3:2:3:2. Le rapport cis/trans est d'environ deux tiers, les isomères 1R et 1S étant présents en quantités égales (racémique). C'est l'isomère [1R,cis] qui est l'insecticide le plus actif; vient ensuite l'isomère [1R,trans].

La perméthrine de qualité technique se présente sous la forme d'un liquide brun ou brun jaunâtre qui peut partiellement cristalliser à la température ambiante. Son point de fusion est d'environ 35°C et son point d'ébullition de 220°C sous 0,05 mmHg. La densité est de 1,214 à 25°C et la tension de vapeur de 1,3 μPa à 20°C. La perméthrine est pratiquement insoluble dans l'eau (moins de 0,2 mg par litre à 25°C), mais elle est soluble dans certains solvants organiques tels que l'acétone, l'hexane et le xylène. Elle est stable à la lumière et à la chaleur, mais instable en milieu alcalin.

Le dosage des résidus et les analyses écotoxicologiques s'effectuent par chromatographie en phase gazeuse avec détection par capture d'électrons (concentration minimale décelable de 0,005 mg/kg). Pour l'analyse des produits techniques, on a recours à la chromatographie en phase gazeuse avec détection par ionisation de flamme.

1.2 Production et usage

On utilise actuellement dans le monde environ 600 tonnes de perméthrine par an, essentiellement en agriculture. Ce produit pourrait être utilisé pour la protection des céréales ensilées et on l'emploie en épandage aérien pour la protection des forêts, la lutte anti-vectorielle, la destruction des insectes incommodants dans les habitations, le déparasitage des bestiaux, la destruction des poux du corps et l'imprégnation des moustiquaires.

La perméthrine est présentée en concentré émulsionnable, en concentré pour application à très bas volume, en poudre mouillable, en poudre pour poudrage et en aérosols.

1.3 Exposition humaine

Les teneurs en résidus des diverses récoltes diminuent assez lentement, le temps de demi-élimination allant de une à trois semaines selon les plantes. Toutefois, lorsqu'elle est utilisée conformément aux recommandations, la perméthrine ne donne pas lieu à une accumulation de résidus, même après plusieurs traitements.

Pour ce qui est de la population dans son ensemble, la voie d'exposition à la perméthrine est essentiellement alimentaire. Les taux de résidus dans les plantes correctement cultivées sont généralement faibles. L'exposition qui pourrait en résulter pour la population générale est vraisemblablement faible, mais on manque de données précises provenant d'études sur la ration totale.

On est très peu documenté sur l'exposition professionnelle à la perméthrine.

1.4 Destinée dans l'environnement

On a montré en laboratoire que la perméthrine se dégrade dans le sol avec une demi-vie d'environ 28 jours. L'isomère trans se décompose plus rapidement que l'isomère cis, la principale réaction de décomposition initiale étant le clivage du groupement ester. Cette réaction donne naissance à des composés qui subissent une oxydation plus poussée aboutissant à l'anhydride carbonique comme produit final. On a montré, en étudiant le potentiel de lessivage de la perméthrine et de ses produits de dégradation, que toutes ces substances pénétraient peu profondément dans le sol.

La perméthrine déposée sur les végétaux se dégrade avec une demi-vie d'environ 10 jours. La principale voie de dégradation comporte le clivage du groupement ester et la conjugaison de l'acide et de l'alcool qui en résultent. Il se produit également une hydroxylation en divers points de la molécule ainsi qu'une interconversion cis-trans photo-induite.

Dans l'eau et à la surface du sol, la perméthrine est décomposée par le rayonnement solaire. Là encore, le clivage du groupement ester et l'interconversion cis-trans sont les principales réactions.

En général, ce processus de décomposition environnementale conduit à des produits de moindre toxicité.

La perméthrine disparaît rapidement de l'environnement, en six à 24 heures dans les étangs et les cours d'eau, en sept jours dans les sédiments des étangs, et en 58 jours dans les feuilles et le sol des forêts. On a constaté que 30% du composé disparaissaient en une semaine des feuilles d'une plantation de cotonniers.

En conditions d'aérobiose dans le sol, la perméthrine se décompose avec une demi-vie de 28 jours.

La perméthrine se déplace peu dans l'environnement et il est improbable qu'elle s'y accumule en quantité notable.

1.5 Cinétique et métabolisme

Administrée à des mammifères, la perméthrine est rapidement métabolisée et presqu'entièrement excrétée dans les urines et les matières fécales en l'espace de 12 jours. L'isomère trans, beaucoup plus sensible à l'attaque par l'estérase que l'isomère cis, s'élimine plus rapidement que ce dernier. Les principales réactions métaboliques sont le clivage du groupement ester et l'oxydation, particulièrement au niveau du cycle aromatique terminal, du reste phénoxybenzylique et du groupe diméthyle géminé du cycle cyclopropane, réactions qui sont suivies d'une conjugaison. On a retrouvé moins de 0,7% de la dose initiale dans le lait de chèvres et de vaches à qui l'on avait administré de la perméthrine par voie orale.

1.6 Effets sur les êtres vivants dans leur milieu naturel

Des épreuves de laboratoire ont montré que la perméthrine était extrêmement toxique pour les arthropodes aquatiques, la CL_{50} allant de 0,018 μg/litre pour la larve d'un crabe comestible à 1,26 μg/litre pour un cladocère. Elle est également très toxique pour les poissons, la CL_{50} à 96 heures allant de 0,62 μg/litre pour la larve de truite arc-en-ciel à 314 μg/litre pour la truite adulte. La dose sans effet observable au début du cycle évolutif du vairon est 10 μg/litre sur 28 jours, la dose chronique étant de 0,66 à 1,4 μg/litre pour un autre cyprinidé, *Pimephas promelas*. La perméthrine est moins toxique pour les mollusques aquatiques et les amphibiens, les valeurs de la CL_{50} à 96 heures se situant respectivement à plus de 1000 μg/litre et 7000 μg/litre.

Lors d'essais sur le terrain et en utilisation normale, cette forte toxicité potentielle ne se manifeste pas. Il existe une abondante littérature sur les effets de la perméthrine utilisée en agriculture, dans les exploitations forestières ainsi que pour la lutte antivectorielle dans de nombreuses régions du monde. Il y a une certaine mortalité pour les arthropodes aquatiques, notamment lorsque l'on traite les eaux en surface, mais les effets sur les populations ne sont que temporaires. Il n'y a pas eu de cas de mortalité chez les poissons. Cette moindre toxicité qui se manifeste sur le terrain provient de la forte adsorption du composé par les sédiments et de sa décomposition rapide.

La perméthrine fixée sur les sédiments est toxique pour les organismes fouisseurs, mais là encore, l'effet est temporaire. La perméthrine est extrêmement toxique pour les abeilles. La DL_{50} topique est de 0,11 μg par abeille mais le fort effet répulsif qu'elle exerce sur l'insecte en réduit les effets toxiques dans la pratique. Rien n'indique qu'il puisse y avoir une forte mortalité des abeilles en utilisation normale. La perméthrine est plus toxique pour les acariens prédateurs que pour les espèces nuisibles visées.

La perméthrine est très peu toxique pour les oiseaux, en administration orale ou par voie alimentaire. La DL_{50} aiguë est supérieure à 3000 mg par kg de poids corporel en une seule administration et supérieure à 5000 mg par kg de nourriture quand le produit est mêlé à la ration. Elle n'a aucun effet sur la reproduction de la poule à la dose de 40 mg/kg de nourriture.

Les organismes aquatiques accumulent facilement la perméthrine, le facteur de concentration allant de 43 à 750 selon les espèces. Chez tous les organismes aquatiques étudiés, la perméthrine disparaît rapidement lorsque les animaux sont remis en eau propre. Il n'y a aucune accumulation chez les oiseaux. On peut donc considérer que ce composé ne présente en pratique aucune tendance à la bioaccumulation.

1.7 Effets sur les animaux d'expérience et sur les systèmes d'épreuve *in vitro.*

La perméthrine n'a qu'une faible toxicité aiguë pour les rats, les souris, les lapins et les cobayes, encore que la DL_{50} varie considérablement selon le véhicule utilisé et le rapport des isomères cis/trans. Les signes d'intoxication aiguë apparaissent en deux heures et persistent jusqu'à trois jours. Les isomères [1R,cis] et [1R,trans] appartiennent aux pyréthroïdes du type-I dont les effets caractéristiques sont les tremblements (syndrome T) la perte de coordination, l'hyperactivité, la prostration et la paralysie. L'intoxication provoque une augmentation notable de la température centrale.

Aucun des métabolites de la perméthrine ne présente une toxicité aiguë (par voie orale ou intrapéritonéale) supérieure à celle de la perméthrine elle-même.

La perméthrine a provoqué une légère irritation de la peau intacte ou abrasée chez le lapin, mais il n'y a pas eu d'irritation d'origine photochimique après exposition aux rayons ultra-violets de zones de la peau traitées par cet insecticide. Elle ne suscite en revanche aucune réaction de sensibilisation chez le cobaye.

Des études de toxicité orale subaiguë et subchronique ont été effectuées chez le rat et la souris à des doses allant jusqu'à 10 000 mg/kg de nourriture et pendant des périodes s'étendant de 14 à 26 semaines. A la dose la plus forte, on a observé une augmentation du rapport poids du foie/poids du corps, une hypertrophie du foie et des signes cliniques d'intoxication tels que des tremblements. Chez le rat, la dose sans effet observable varie de 20 mg/kg de nourriture (pour les études de 90 jours ou de six mois) à 150 mg/kg de nourriture (lors d'une étude de six mois).

Chez le chien, ces valeurs ont été trouvées égales à 50 mg/kg de poids corporel et à 100 mg/kg de poids corporel, respectivement, lors de deux études de trois mois.

Des études à long terme sur des souris et des rats ont révélé une augmentation du poids du foie, vraisemblablement liée à l'induction du système enzymatique des microsomes hépatiques.

Une étude de deux ans sur des rats a fait ressortir une dose sans effet observable de 100 mg/kg de nourriture, soit 5 mg/kg de poids corporel.

D'après trois études à long terme sur la souris, il semblerait qu'il existe un certain pouvoir cancérogène au niveau des poumons pour au moins une souche de souris (uniquement des femelles) à la dose la plus élevée étudiée, soit 5 g/kg de nourriture. Aucun effet oncogène n'a été observé chez des rats des deux sexes.

La perméthrine n'est mutagène ni *in vivo* ni *in vitro*.

Les études de mutagénicité ainsi que des études à long terme sur la souris et le rat indiquent que le pouvoir oncogène de la perméthrine est très faible, qu'il se limite aux souris femelles et qu'il s'agit probablement d'un phénomène épigénétique.

La perméthrine n'est pas tératogène pour le rat, la souris ou le lapin, à des doses allant respectivement jusqu'à 225, 150 et 1800 mg/kg de poids corporel.

La perméthrine n'a pas produit d'effet indésirable à des doses allant jusqu'à 2500 mg/kg de nourriture lors d'une étude de reproduction portant sur trois générations.

Administrée à des rats à forte dose (6600 à 7000 mg/kg de nourriture) pendant 14 jours, l'insecticide a provoqué des lésions au niveau du nerf sciatique; cependant une autre étude n'a pas confirmé la présence d'altérations ultrastructurales à ce niveau. Chez la poule on n'a pas observé de neurotoxicité retardée.

1.8 Effets sur l'homme

La perméthrine peut provoquer un certain nombre de sensations au niveau de la peau ainsi que des paresthésies chez les travailleurs exposés, symptômes qui apparaissent après une période de latence d'environ 30 minutes, passent par un maximum au bout de huit heures et disparaissent en 24 heures. Parmi les symptômes les plus fréquemment signalés, figurent un engourdissement, des démangeaisons, des fourmillements et des sensations de brûlure.

Aucun cas d'intoxication n'a été signalé.

La probabilité d'effets oncogènes chez l'homme est extrêmement faible, voire nulle.

Rien n'indique que la perméthrine puisse exercer des effets indésirables sur l'homme si elle est utilisée conformément aux recommandations.

2. Conclusions

2.1 Population générale

La population dans son ensemble est vraisemblablement très peu exposée à la perméthrine. Cet insecticide ne devrait présenter aucun danger s'il est utilisé conformément aux recommandations.

2.2 Exposition professionnelle

Utilisée de manière raisonnable et moyennant certaines mesures d'hygiène et de sécurité, la perméthrine ne devrait présenter aucun danger pour les personnes qui lui sont exposées de par leur profession.

2.3 Environnement

La perméthrine ou ses produits de décomposition ne devraient pas atteindre dans le milieu des concentrations critiques dans la mesure où l'insecticide est utilisé aux doses recommandées. Au laboratoire, la perméthrine est extrêmement toxique pour les poissons, les arthropodes aquatiques et les abeilles. Toutefois il est improbable que des effets indésirables durables se produisent en situation réelle si l'insecticide est utilisé conformément aux recommandations.

3. Recommandations

Les concentrations alimentaires résultant d'une utilisation conforme aux recommandations sont en principe faibles, toutefois il serait bon de confirmer cette hypothèse en étendant la surveillance à la perméthrine.

La perméthrine est utilisée depuis de nombreuses années sans qu'aucun effet indésirable n'ait été signalé à la suite d'une exposition humaine. Néanmoins il serait bon de poursuivre les observations sur ce type d'exposition.

